Doctor, What if it Were Your Mother?

*Hope, Faith and Reason
at the End of Life*

Victor G. Vogel, MD

Copyright © 2014 Victor G. Vogel.

All rights reserved. No part of this book may be used or reproduced by any means, graphic, electronic, or mechanical, including photocopying, recording, taping or by any information storage retrieval system without the written permission of the publisher except in the case of brief quotations embodied in critical articles and reviews.

All Bible verses quoted are from The Holy Bible, New International Version®, NIV® Copyright © 1973, 1978, 1984, 2011 by Biblica, Inc.® Used by permission. All rights reserved worldwide.

WestBow Press books may be ordered through booksellers or by contacting:

WestBow Press
A Division of Thomas Nelson & Zondervan
1663 Liberty Drive
Bloomington, IN 47403
www.westbowpress.com
1 (866) 928-1240

Because of the dynamic nature of the Internet, any web addresses or links contained in this book may have changed since publication and may no longer be valid. The views expressed in this work are solely those of the author and do not necessarily reflect the views of the publisher, and the publisher hereby disclaims any responsibility for them.

Any people depicted in stock imagery provided by Thinkstock are models, and such images are being used for illustrative purposes only. Certain stock imagery © Thinkstock.

ISBN: 978-1-4908-5589-9 (sc)
ISBN: 978-1-4908-5591-2 (hc)
ISBN: 978-1-4908-5590-5 (e)

Library of Congress Control Number: 2014918302

Printed in the United States of America.

WestBow Press rev. date: 11/10/2014

Contents

Introduction vii

1. Rendezvous with Death 1
2. The First Time: Death of a Friend 12
3. Can You Save Him, Doc? 28
4. Understanding Suffering Through Reason 44
5. Defeating Death for a Time 62
6. Lifeguard: Death in the Family 84
7. Through a Glass Darkly 100
8. Death Stops for Me 115
9. A Bulwark Never Failing 134
10. Faith, Reason, and Suffering with Technology 153
11. We Happy Few: Sharing Grief with Friends 173
12. Contemplating Suffering and Doubt from a Distance 187
13. A Christian Perspective on Suffering and Death ... 202
14. Lessons from My Patients: Grace Within Suffering 217
15. Resolving Grief through Service to Others 231
16. Some Thoughts on Grace 255
17. The Spiritual Challenge of Sharing Bad News 264
18. Hope and Futility: What if it Were Your Mother? 281
19. Some Final Thoughts on Communicating Hope 310

Acknowledgments 323
Biography 329

Introduction

> One's experience becomes visible when given form. Experience without mediation through representation is evanescent, not because it's forgotten, but because without material form—painting, story, poem—it cannot be beheld, and so it's as if it never happened.[1]
> —R. Charon

All adults will face suffering, grief, and loss in their own lives and in the lives of the people they love. They will want to offer hope and comfort to those who are dying and to respond compassionately to the needs of their friends and family. The purpose of this book is to use examples from my life and experience as a Christian physician who relies on his faith in his daily practice to show how grief can be overcome and how family and friends can best minister to the sick and dying. I also show how very sick and dying patients can make rational decisions to assure that they receive the most compassionate and effective care. Finally, I show how service to others can be a cure for grief and loss.

When doctors are blunt and specific about prognosis, patients sometimes perceive this as removing or destroying hope, but all mortal life ends eventually. At some point, each of us must confront the reality of our individual mortality, the certainty that we will die. It is always appropriate for physicians to look for effective cures for those afflictions that are amenable to therapy, but a mortal end awaits all of us. Hope arises both from knowing that our doctors will alleviate or delay our suffering, to be sure, but our ultimate hope comes from knowing, through faith alone, that when we die, we will not die into eternal loneliness, separation, anxiety, torture, or damnation. Rather, we will pass from death to life, and thereby into the loving, comforting, and abiding presence of our immortal God. From that knowledge comes our surest hope and comfort.

My assurance to the doubter, the skeptic, and the nonbeliever is that I know this for them even if they cannot or will not believe it themselves. My hope for them can generate hope in them, even if their hope is merely temporal or is only in me and my treatments. Hope in a quiet death and hope for a quiet exit is hope, indeed, even if my patient cannot hope for or find reassurance in eternal things.

This book describes how I, as a medical oncologist, have dealt with personal suffering, pain, and loss, the death of my family members, and the deaths of my patients during a thirty-year career of caring for people with cancer and other serious medical illnesses. I describe how to support and sustain patients and their families through troubling emotion, grief, and loss, and I identify skills to help all of us die with grace and hope. I show caregivers and patients how to remain honest and engaged and how to offer affirming support that celebrates the life of the person who is dying.

The book is illustrated with examples and lessons that I have learned from my personal illnesses and accidents. It also contains actual stories about my patients who have died (and some who have survived) under my care. I explain how individuals in both my family and my medical practices have maintained hope and optimism until the end. I have tried to illustrate these stories with both compassion and honesty to show how objectivity and rational medical decision making can ultimately bring the greatest comfort to those who are dying. I show what can be done when curative medicine fails to bring about the desired result, and I offer a Christian apologetic to answer the most difficult question: "Why does a loving God allow us to suffer and die?" I also explain why faith is the foundation of hope and how faith can inform difficult medical decision making at the end of life. I try to offer practical solutions to grief and longing and to describe the urgent need in American medicine for more care that is delivered with palliative, rather than curative, intent as a generation of baby boomers confronts increasingly challenging decisions for our parents and, ultimately, for ourselves in the face of constantly rising health care costs.

This is not a book about faith healing or spiritual counseling, nor do I espouse euthanasia or mercy killing. There is a large and growing literature on these topics, and I will not attempt to improve on them or expand the scope of their coverage here.[2] This is, rather, a book of personal stories, of real clinical and personal experiences that I have had during a thirty-year medical career as a general internist, as an academic clinical researcher, as a practicing medical oncologist, and as a patient who experienced a life-threatening injury at a very young age. I have also participated in the deaths of dear family members, including my mother, who died from acute leukemia at the age of sixty-three. All of these experiences have influenced deeply the way in which I regard, encounter, and manage illness, suffering, and death in my patients. Because I am a medical oncologist, dying patients are, sadly, not strangers to me. In this book, I recount their stories and what I have learned from them.

I have been a Christian all of my adult life. I was confirmed by my father, a Protestant pastor, when I was a young teenager. I am a Presbyterian elder and a member of the board of directors of the Pittsburgh Theological Seminary. I have at times been a professing Methodist and a Lutheran, and I regard myself as a typical or usual mainline Protestant church member in the early twenty-first century. I am not a mystic, and I do not practice what some would refer to as "faith healing." I do not pray with my patients, and I did not evangelize to them. I am not a medical missionary, and I am not ordained as a lay pastor. I do, however, have a deep and profound faith in God. I have studied my faith, questioned it, doubted it, examined it, argued about it, defended it, and ultimately came to love it as a source of real comfort and clarity as I wrestled with the intensely disturbing suffering and loss that I witness every day in my patients and occasionally in my own life and in the lives of those whom I love.

I cannot ultimately answer the deep spiritual questions about where God is when we suffer or why we suffer, but I believe that he is always present in our suffering. I believe, too, that God participates in our personal suffering and loss in ways that we cannot fully know or adequately comprehend. My father often spoke about God's blessings both known and unknown. This faith in his perpetual, ineluctable presence during illness has given me an optimism and hope during serious illness that I have tried to portray to and share with my patients. I have attempted to explain some of this in this book.

I do not condone and have never practiced active euthanasia (although I have witnessed it), and I do not discuss its few merits and many great faults in this book. Neither do I condone forgoing medical therapy when it offers the potential for cure. Disappointingly, however, we have many situations in clinical medicine—those best known to me are from medical oncology—where prudence would often dictate that we seek palliative rather than curative interventions for our patients. Sadly, too, available data indicate that we do not do this nearly often enough in American medical clinics and hospitals.

There are multiple causes of this failure of our system to care appropriately for those who are dying. There is much evidence to support the contention that the major fault lies with us physicians and not so much with our patients. To be sure, both patients and physicians have access to a great deal of information, and many medical specialists are blessed with new, active therapies that can sometimes cure or very often prolong the lives of our patients who are afflicted with life-threatening illnesses. The data show, however, that American physicians and their patients do not know what to say when the end has arrived and a patient should be allowed to die in peace.[3] I examine our limitations herein and offer some alternatives to our currently inadequate practices.

We now have medications in medical oncology that cost thousands of dollars per month, hundreds of thousands of dollars per year, and that increase the time before death by only two to three months;[4] then, mournfully and predictably, the patient dies. Do such therapies add meaningfully to the lives of these patients and their families? Does the use of such medication divert us from addressing and dealing with the deeper and more profound questions with which our patients and their loved ones are struggling? Has our technologically based medicine replaced our opportunity to truly care for our patients as they die?

Our failing here is by and with us physicians who communicate poorly with our patients about realistic expectations and outcomes from our therapies. We physicians do badly, apparently, at conveying a prognosis when it is very poor or fatal, and many patients have been conditioned to believe that hope comes only through the use of therapeutic interventions (such as surgery, medical devices, medications, and procedures) and not from spiritual reflection and wrestling with life's most deep and profound questions. We lack the realization that hope lies as often in our caring as in our curing.

What I illustrate in this book is that hope can come from optimism that arises out of faith. I do not propose that patients or the public adopt my particular beliefs. Rather, I discuss the tenets of my faith as an example of a belief system that gives me comfort, helps me to explain suffering, offers hope in illness and death, and supports decision making that embraces palliative approaches to life-threatening illness when such approaches are appropriate.

Faith and spirituality have been marginalized in much of clinical medicine even though the majority of Americans espouse a belief in God and say that spirituality should be included in their care. Faith in God, who participates in our suffering and promises life beyond death, will lead to different decisions if patients are given a chance to exercise choices based on faith and hope. I will not argue that my faith should be imposed on the nonbeliever or the skeptic, nor am I advocating that we ration care. I argue, rather, that a communication strategy that seeks to educate patients and their families about realistic expectations that arise from limited therapies in the face of life-threatening illness will lead them to make different decisions than they would make in the absence of such communication.

When I was a medical oncology fellow at Johns Hopkins thirty years ago, there was a young woman whom I shall call Jennifer who had been treated for acute leukemia and had relapsed twice after her treatments, which included a bone marrow transplantation. The hematologists and oncologists who were taking care of Jennifer believed that it was futile to attempt to treat her leukemia for a third time with yet another round of induction therapy, because available data showed that it was extremely unlikely that additional therapy would be successful. Unfortunately, this young woman eventually succumbed to her disease.

Despite our urgings for Jennifer to initiate best supportive care during her remaining days, she was adamant that we treat her with another round of anti-leukemic chemotherapy. In exasperation, the medical team caring for Jennifer consulted the director of the hospital chaplaincy service, the Reverend Clyde Shallenberger, to help us explore with Jennifer her reasons for demanding additional treatment. For years, the Reverend Shallenberger had overseen an annual educational event originally called the Institute on Ministry with the Sick at Johns Hopkins (now known as the Institute for Spirituality and Medicine). Clyde had a reputation for being both thoughtful and compassionate in his dealings with patients and families who faced difficult medical and ethical decisions in the hospital.

The medical oncology attending physician, the Reverend Shallenberger, several nurses, and I met with Jennifer in her hospital room one morning after rounds. The Reverend Shallenberger compassionately explored with Jennifer what she knew about her diagnosis, its prior treatment, and her prognosis. He gently but persistently inquired of Jennifer why it was so important to her that she receive additional therapy. After several cautious and evasive answers, Jennifer exclaimed with flowing tears and much emotion, "If I don't get treated again, my family will think I am a failure!" Our team lovingly reassured her that such a decision would not in any way reflect cowardice, lack of conviction, or a failure by her. With a sense of mutual resolution, both Jennifer and her family agreed after our meeting that we would not give her additional anti-leukemia treatment. She died quietly at home a few weeks later while receiving supportive hospice care with her family at her side.

Doctors and patients must both confront and wrestle with the reality of their own mortality. Only when we have settled in our own souls that we will die can we be at peace with ourselves. Only then can we hope to help others who are suffering. I realize that not everyone comes to a spiritual answer to apprehensions about their mortality, but all must come to an objective understanding that we will die. I believe that denial of death has led to irrational treatments and unrealistic expectations, and that these expectations are engendered and aggravated by poor doctor-patient communication that can be overcome.

I will discuss strategies for improving communication between doctors and patients. I will show examples of how I have shared bad news with my patients and with my family when we confronted serious illness together. I will show what I have learned about what patients want, and how that knowledge can be translated into comforting, palliative care at the end of life while always maintaining hope.

---

[1] Charon, R. The reciprocity of recognition—What medicine exposes about self and other. *N Engl J Med* 2012;367:1878–1881.

2. Puchalski, Christina M., and Ferrell, Betty. *Making Health Care Whole: Integrating Spirituality into Patient Care.* West Conshohocken, PA: Templeton Press, 2010.
3. See, for example, Puchalski, Christina MA. *Time for Listening and Caring: spirituality and the care of the chronically ill and dying.* New York: Oxford University Press, 2006.
4. Cortes J, O'Shaughnessy J, Loesch D, et al. Erubulin monotherapy versus treatment of physician's choice in patients with metastatic breast cancer (EMBRACE): a phase 3 open-label randomized study. *Lancet* 2011;377:914–923.

1

Rendezvous with Death

> I have a rendezvous with Death At some disputed barricade, When Spring comes back with rustling shade And apple-blossoms fill the air—[1]
> —Alan Seeger

Doctors learn about death through their clinical training in medical school, from teaching by their mentors, and through their training as residents and interns in their specialty after medical school. Rarely, we come very close to it through a personal encounter with illness or injury.

As a child, I was quite fond of cold weather. Maybe it was a vestige of my German heritage. The winter Olympics intrigued me at a young age, and I tried to blacken my mother's white ice skates with liquid polish before I wore them at the neighborhood pond (we couldn't afford a pair of boys' skates for me for several years). My hockey stick had a roll of electrical tape on the blade to keep it from breaking. When the snow fell and the temperature dropped, I was drawn outside on weekends because Sunday afternoons at my house were always a little too quiet for my liking. Either my parents were taking naps, or Dad was out on church business, and winter afternoons were quiet and boring. Like most youngsters, I sought adventure. It is not clear now, years later, how I was given quite so much freedom at six years of age, but I recall being able to explore the neighborhood alone.

Our Lightning Glider sled had been a Christmas present to the family. My sister, Louise, never showed much interest in it, and my brother Tim, at age three, couldn't handle it by himself. Our house in east York was on the edge of a growing city where suburban housing development met rich Pennsylvania farmland. The land was crossed by streams winding through gentle, rolling hills that provided endless adventure for a young explorer. The January day was pleasantly cold. I could see out my bedroom window through the backyard to the hill at the neighbor's yard about a quarter mile away where many children and a few adults were having a giggling, shouting time sledding on the steep hill. The activity on the hill called me that afternoon, but I knew that if I joined the fun, I would be alone. Mom wouldn't want to bring my brother and sister along, and Dad was visiting a TWA captain and his wife on a pastoral call. Waiting until he came home did not seem an attractive alternative. I also knew that once I arrived on the hill, there would be plenty of companionship.

Mother gave assent to my request to join the sledding, simply asking that I be in by dark. I quickly donned snowsuit and boots, hat and mittens, and was off across the yards. It was a short walk, and the closer I got, the more I could hear the delighted yells of children gliding down the steep hill. The sledding trail was a straight path that began at the back of a house atop the hill. The top half of the run was a bit treacherous, because on the right side, about a hundred feet down, was a sheer drop of twenty feet where a level area to make a garden had been cut into the hill by the property owner below. Beyond this, the path narrowed, flanked by another garden on the left and trees and shrubs on the right. At the bottom, the track widened as the upper yard and garden joined the yard of the house at the bottom of the hill. The only obstacles at the bottom were three widely spaced metal wash-line poles anchored in concrete at the back of the house that marked the base of the track. The entire run was about two hundred yards long with a drop of about eighty feet that produced a manageable course and quite an exciting ride.

Manageable, that is, without ice on the surface. The hill had seen quite a bit of activity that afternoon, and the repeated trips by sled runners going down the hill combined with feet treading back up the hill had made a tightly packed, slick surface. In midafternoon—when the hill was at peak activity—the sun was warm, and the snow was soft and wet in places. Even toboggans negotiated the hill with little difficulty. Later in the afternoon, though, as the crowd wore thin and the sun began to slide behind the crest of the eastward-looking hill, the slick surface became frozen hard. With lengthening shadows and a growing chill, there were few people left on the hill by late afternoon.

I negotiated many runs down the incline that afternoon without incident. Once, I did slide near the top, and the front of my sled delivered a glancing blow to the leg of a friend plodding slowly up the hill. He yelled when I hit him, but even more so when he fell down the cut near the top of the run. He shouted something about being careful and trudged slowly home, alternately bawling at me and sobbing as he went. I was sorry for having ended his day, but I hadn't done it intentionally; it seemed to be one of those acceptable hazards of the hill. It was also an omen.

The trips later in the afternoon were, in many ways, more fun because the speed was faster. In another way, they were less of a challenge because the hill was not as crowded and there were fewer people to avoid as I careened toward the bottom. I really had not thought much about quitting for the day when I began what was to be my last run. I wasn't cold, and even though the long shadows of the late winter afternoon belied the approaching darkness, there was still plenty of daylight. I flopped belly down on my sled at the top, and because of the excessive incline, gathered speed quickly. I recall very little of the ride to the bottom, except that I was going very fast. I negotiated the narrow path between the bushes and the garden without difficulty, but as soon as I burst out into the wide area where I had stopped successfully earlier, I knew I was in trouble.

Most runs that afternoon had ended with a loss of momentum at the bottom of the hill, but now the house appeared to be approaching very fast, and its concrete foundation loomed ominously beneath its wooden siding. Were I doing that run again now, I would roll off the sled. At the time, the sled seemed too secure, too friendly to abandon. To avoid hitting the house straight on at great speed, I pulled back as hard as I could on the right handle, thinking that, at worst, the side of the sled would strike the house and absorb the blow. What my six-year-old mind could not anticipate was that I would be flung to the outside of the ensuing turn by the centrifugal force induced by the abrupt change of direction that occurred at high speed. With the sudden turn, I entered an uncontrolled slide to my left while in the slow right turn. I was moving too fast to be afraid, and in an instant, I knew I would miss the house.

But my accelerated skid had not yet ended, and my exposed left flank struck one of the anchored metal wash-line poles with full force, stopping the sled abruptly. I immediately vomited in the snow while rolling off the sled to my right in severe pain. As I lay groaning on the cold, snow-covered lawn, two much older boys arrived from the hill and asked what had happened. I agonizingly explained while shedding no tears. They knew who I was, and they assured me they would take me home on the sled.

I remember nothing of that ride home.

My mother's response when we arrived at our back door is vivid in my memory, however. She was neither frantic nor hysterical. She was a nurse, and through all types of adversity, I had never seen her lose her composure. Miraculously, I struggled into the house while the boys were explaining the mishap. Neither of the boys thought that I was seriously hurt, and one even reported that supposed fact to his mother. Inside my house, it did not take me long to realize that my mother was quite concerned. She later told me that I looked terribly pale, and I can remember not wanting to move from my recumbent position on the living room couch. With each passing minute, the pain in my abdomen increased, and I gingerly held my left side.

My father arrived home in a short time, within an hour of my arrival, and engaged in muffled discussions with my mother in the kitchen. I could hear them making telephone calls. I later learned that one was to our family doctor to schedule an urgent examination. Another was to arrange babysitting for my seven-year-old sister and three-year-old brother. That accomplished, I was loaded into the rear seat of our gray 1952 Chevy, which still had snow chains on the rear tires. The first few miles were quite uncomfortable for me because of the vibration of the chains on the bare roads and highway that only aggravated my tender belly even more. The first stop was at a service station, where the chains were quickly removed.

The next thing I recall is being examined by Dr. George Gardner, our family physician. His office was at his home, which seems curious years later, but perhaps not nearly as curious as seeing him at six o'clock on a Sunday evening. By the time we arrived at his office, I was weak and lightheaded. Dr. Gardner was a quiet man, but even quieter this night. His attention was focused on my abdomen that by now was quite tender to his gently probing hand. He kept poking under my ribs on the left, and after a few minutes I was nauseated. He held a hushed conference with my parents in a corner of the examining room; it was the first indication other than my pain that something serious was evolving.

My mother approached the examining table and said that we would have to go to the hospital. I was too weak to protest. The four-mile trip from Dr. Gardner's office to the hospital was a blur, and with each passing mile and each evolving minute, I was getting sicker. It seems curious in retrospect that we did not use an ambulance. On our arrival, a hospital orderly met us with a wheelchair that Dr. Gardner had ordered. My father and the orderly lifted me out of the car and wheeled me into an emergency room cubicle, where they placed me on a stretcher. No matter how I turned, I could not relieve the growing pain.

I now realize that I was in early physiological shock, and over a period of a few minutes, I was progressively overwhelmed by an urgent need to defecate. For reasons that remain unclear to this day—and ignoring most rules for dealing with incipient shock—the orderly took me off the stretcher and put me on a bedpan on the seat of the wheelchair. My mother was not happy with the decision because she herself had placed many bedpans under many patients lying in their beds. Out of deference to the orderly, however, she stood by nervously as I slumped painfully in the wheelchair.

At that instant I began to slip off into unconsciousness, but a loud and authoritative voice shattered the silence.

"Get that boy onto a stretcher!" shouted Wesley Dehaven Stick, staff surgeon at York Hospital.

What moments before had been chaos now became a tense calm. The orderly and my mother rapidly put me back on the stretcher. Years later, as I examined patients in shock whose eyes were glassy and rolled upward, whose skin was dull and cool with the perspiration that accompanies adrenaline excess, I knew what they must be feeling. The world gets very narrow in your perception as blood pressure falls, and thoughts are focused only on the pain. All your hopes and fears are focused on and transferred to your physician. Whereas Dr. Gardner had been gentle and concerned, Dr. Stick was firm and decisive. After his rapid exam, another hushed conversation with my parents was followed by my mother earnestly explaining an operation to me. It seemed that I had ruptured my spleen with the sudden impact against the wash-line pole. I was annoyed with the simplistic clarification that an operation meant "cutting my tummy." At the same time, I wondered what a spleen was, and no one seemed to have a satisfactory explanation. I never had a chance to ask Dr. Stick.

I was to learn subsequently that he was habitually too rushed to answer my questions, and I was so intimidated by his decisiveness and authority that I was usually unable to frame my questions adequately before he had left my bedside. I would wait fifteen years for a thorough explanation of splenic anatomy and physiology, which came, ironically, as I watched a splenectomy for the first time during my undergraduate work/study program at a Baltimore hospital.

I experienced quite a few emotions that evening, but fear was not one of them. On hearing that a trip to the operating room was to follow urgently, I was not terrified. For me, this had become a journey of wonderment and adventure. It was as though a cave had opened at the bottom of that icy hill, and exploring it was more exhilarating than all the rides down that treacherous slope earlier in the afternoon. It was a great help that I did not appreciate the danger I faced. Accurate knowledge about just how sick I was surely would have blunted my boyish excitement and inquisitiveness.

I can recite most of the ensuing events not from memory but from supposition based on what I now know must have occurred. Most of the details are not relevant, however, with two exceptions. At some time in the emergency room, an intravenous line was inserted into my arm. A transfusion of whole blood quickly followed the saline infusion. I cannot recall pain or discomfort from any of the venipunctures. My only memory is of the trip to the operating room. A male orderly pushed my gurney feet-first down the hall from behind my head. At my side, a nurse held the glass bottle that contained the blood being transfused into my arm high over her head. There was no pole on which to hang the bottle, which is curious in retrospect. The glass bottle seems even more anachronistic. (This was the late 1950s, before plastics transformed virtually every routine in clinical medicine.)

As we wheeled past green tile walls, the hallways had a darkened, eerie silence, and I was very much alone for the first time in my life. Perhaps these strangers sensed my loneliness, or perhaps they were fearful for me, wondering why a six-year-old showed so little concern. Whatever their reasons, they were somewhat jovial. I have since mused that they were lovers, but I doubt it was so. As we moved along, they chatted idly and nervously as I listened anxiously.

Then the nurse said suddenly to the orderly, "If you say that I look like the Statue of Liberty, I'll break this bottle over your head!"

"Don't do that!" I pleaded, and we all laughed. I knew they were not serious; I wonder if they knew that I was.

The operating room was enchantingly mysterious. Never before in my very young life had I seen such concealed wonder. I had found the excitement I was searching for earlier in the afternoon. It was as though I had been ushered into the inner sanctum of a forbidden world. I wanted to leap off the gurney and explore to my heart's content, but masked women speaking in muffled tones were intent on directing my movements. The masks only added to the intrigue. I could sense that I was getting drowsy, but the pain in my abdomen was also subsiding. I wondered where Dr. Stick was and what he was doing, and I wondered what all the gadgets were for. My eyes were being bathed in a flood of new sights, and I wanted to look, and explore, and question, and ...

One of the masked nurses leaned close and said, "Victor, I am going to put this mask on your face, and I want you to breathe normally."

The black rubber anesthesia mask looked like the kind that the fictional US Air Force captain Steve Canyon wore in his jet fighter, so that was fine with me. My brother, Tim, and I slept in US Army surplus wooden bunks at home, and my father had nailed an old board along one side of the top bunk so that I would not drop five feet to the floor in the middle of the night. The other side of the bunk faced the wall, so I was secure. Tim and I used those bunks in our play as everything from covered wagons to jet fighters, and it was the aircraft that I always fantasized about. With a crayon I scratched the words "Victor Vogel—Pilot, Tim Vogel—Copilot" on the rail to leave no doubts in the minds of visitors who trespassed the imagined fantasies of our enchanted room. My chagrinned parents eventually painted both the bunk and the rail. In the middle of the room, plastic aircraft models hung from a string that extended from the ceiling light fixture to the heating vent on the side wall.

As the ether flowed through the mask, I thought of those planes and counted the chunks of calcium carbonate in the glass cylinder next to my head. Then, suddenly, I was flying where not even eagles dared.[2]

They removed three pints of blood along with my spleen from my abdomen that cold January evening. The mother of the boys who brought me home on my sled heard about my injury the next morning on the local radio station. Her sons had told her that I was fine when they brought me home. She called my mother in a panic the next morning, asking if I was all right. Mom assured her that I had survived the accident and the surgery. Mom also told me that the mother of the boys gave them quite a reprimand, although I am not sure why. I never suffered adverse consequences in the ensuing years as a result of the operation, but I had come very close to dying of shock because of blood loss that night. For the first time, I got a glimpse of the enemy and deceiver, death, who would visit my life in many veiled and misleading guises in the decades that followed.

---

[1] "I Have a Rendezvous with Death" by Alan Seeger. *www.poets.org/viewmedia.php/prmMID/19396* (Accessed September 13, 2014)

[2] "Even youths grow tired and weary, and young men stumble and fall; But those who hope in the Lord will renew their strength. They will soar on wings like eagles; they will run and not grow weary, they will walk and not be faint." (Isaiah 40:30–31)

2

The First Time: Death of a Friend

> There is no essence of being, but only infinite being in infinite manifestations. Only an infinitely small part of infinite being comes within my range. The rest of it passes me by, like distant ships to which I make signals they do not understand. But by devoting myself to that which comes within my sphere of influence and needs me, I make spiritual inward devotions to infinite being a reality, and thereby give my own poor existence meaning and richness. The river has found its sea.
> —Albert Schweitzer

I can recall very few encounters with dying patients during medical school, and we had no formal training as medical students about the special needs of those who are dying. I thus arrived at the beginning of my internship, as did many of my colleagues, with little preparation for what we were about to encounter as we cared for dying patients for the first time in our clinical careers.

I had prepared for my postgraduate medical training for eight years, and dreamed about it since adolescence. Internship. Almost a *real* doctor. I had watched *Dr. Kildare* on television every week as a schoolboy and imagined what it was going to be like, dashing about a hospital fighting for patients' lives, warring with chiefs of staff and hospital administrators, and falling in love with a beautiful nurse in my spare time. I was an idealist dreaming of working in glamorous hospitals, admitting, diagnosing, and treating thankful patients.

The allure, anticipation, and excitement of graduating from medical school and embarking on the most dramatic, most challenging, most demanding year of my life as a medical intern soon gave way, however, to a pervading anxiety that was all too real: there was too much to learn in a short time. Certainly, I had been trained to do the job at the Temple University School of Medicine that offers one of the finest clinical educations available in the United States, but as a medical student, there was always the cushion, the safety net that the patients were not really mine. Someone else took the ultimate responsibility if I missed a diagnosis or prescribed the wrong treatment. But now, it was all up to me. No one was looking over my shoulder, no one was there to whom I could shift the burden. Or so I thought.

The Baltimore City Hospitals were founded in 1723 as the Bay View Asylum, a mental institution for the city placed high atop a hill in south-central Baltimore. Looking toward the south from the roof of the new hospital, I could see the steel mills and Baltimore's harbor, through which the ships and commerce of the Eastern Seaboard passed between Baltimore and Norfolk. The community around the hospital had experienced logarithmic growth during World War II, when the wages and the promise of a better life from the steel mill and the shipyard at Sparrows Point attracted workers from the rural south, the Appalachians, and the Midwest. After the war, the area enjoyed continued expanding prosperity for nearly three decades, and the neighborhood grew. This growth, in turn, supported the hospital with a varied and dependable caseload, and much of the community regarded the hospital as "their doctor." They seemed not to mind the regular comings and goings of young physicians who left the institution each June to pursue further training or to practice medicine in another setting. The trainees included surgeons and internists, obstetricians, psychiatrists, pathologists, pediatricians, and radiologists, and a complete cadre of attending staff from all medical subspecialties. The affiliation of the hospital with the Johns Hopkins Medical School and the Hopkins Medical Institutions made it a very attractive training environment, and the list of its residents each year included students from the country's best medical schools.

The training environment could not be called a competitive one in the sense that some of the larger, better-known teaching hospitals in the country are. I never sensed that any of the house staff were trying to outdo each other, and within the limits of everyone's physical and emotional energy, we tried to help each other wherever we could. The problem came with the sheer daily demands of the place. Our lives were grouped into month-long blocks divided by service affiliation. For the internal medicine interns this meant multiple four-week tours in the emergency room, medical wards, and cardiac and intensive care units. Each month was shared with two other interns, a second-year resident, and a senior resident. The interns rotated admitting responsibilities every three days, and admitting days typically involved three to five admissions. In addition to bringing new patients into "the system" on admitting days, the responsibility at night extended to the entire service. At times, this would mean that as many as thirty patients were the responsibility of a single intern in the hospital alone for twelve to fifteen hours. The residents were also in the hospital, somewhere, but the unwritten rule was that unless a life-threatening emergency occurred, the resident would be in bed, and the intern would spend the night taking calls from the nurses about the various needs of the patients.

On a good night, the last admission would arrive on the floor just after dinner, and all the exams and orders would be complete by ten or eleven o'clock. Then there would be two hours or so to take care of minor chores, such as starting new intravenous lines, before going to bed for the night. Even on the best nights, there were calls for various complaints, but many of them could be handled over the telephone. Those were the good nights, and they were rare. On more typical nights the lurking enemy was the crisis that could not be averted, or worse, the crisis in which the intern, through fatigue or stupidity or both, made an error that cost someone their life. These crises happened rarely, but they did occur.

In many ways it was more a forced march in which I was required to maintain a level of physical exertion long after my body could willingly sustain the effort. This was internship, a long, steady, demanding ordeal where the rapid acquisition of crucial technical knowledge was not enough. That knowledge had to be synthesized and categorized and placed into context, ready for recall and future use while, simultaneously, the body executed the daily demands of what, for most interns, became a massive administrative burden. We began each day with "work rounds" when the intern who had been on call the night before presented his or her cases to the rest of the service team so that the next time someone else was on call, they would have a vague idea about the patients and why they were in the hospital. It was also an excellent way to learn from the experience of the other residents. The team visited each patient briefly (usually for no more than five minutes) after which the residents joined the chief of service and the chief resident to report the happenings of the previous day in a colloquy known simply as "Morning Report."

While the residents met with the chiefs, the interns, armed with the advice of the residents from morning rounds, began organizing the day's activities: discharging patients, retrieving results of tests and scheduling new ones, requesting consultations from subspecialty services, and performing routine doctor's duties such as writing orders and prescriptions, writing or dictating admission histories, physical examinations and discharge summaries, and starting new intravenous lines. When time permitted (and attendance was expected), there were conferences and lectures, presentations and reviews, meetings and luncheons. It was learning by mass action, pure and simple. The designers of our training must have felt that if house staff were exposed to important situations often enough in a short period of time, a tremendous transfer of knowledge would, of necessity, occur by the sheer weight of the experience.

Unfortunately, it did not happen that way. In my first six months as an intern, I spent six weeks in the emergency room, eight weeks in the intensive care (ICU) and coronary care (CCU) units, and eight weeks on the medical wards, with a two-week respite on the rheumatology consultation service. By Christmas, I was physically exhausted and at the limits of my emotions. I needed a diversion to preserve my sanity, a physical and emotional release, a true recreation. My wife, Sally, was struggling with her internship during the same time, and we were not very successful at providing emotional support to each other during our years of training. (When we had finally completed eight years of residency and fellowship training as well as our required public service, a friend of ours observed that we were just then "getting married," even though we had already been married nine years when we finally finished our formal education.)

I searched for an activity that would provide recreation and diversion, something that would restore my emotional strength and integrity while offering a skill I could take with me later. I played tennis and I swam and I jogged, but none of that seemed to help in the way that I needed.

Somewhere in my search I told myself I should learn to fly. I am uncertain where the idea arose, what its genesis was, but by the spring of my internship, it was an idea I could not shake. It seemed so attractive, so—well, dashing. I began to read publications about flying. I went to the public library and checked out all the books I could find about flying. It was then that I realized I had read little but science for nine years. I convinced myself that I yearned for something more in my life than just medicine. That admission seemed, in some ways, heretical, because we had been trained to believe that nothing other than medicine mattered. The compulsion began when we were undergraduates and neurotically spent our weekends cramming for exams for which we had already prepared adequately. It continued in medical school when instructors told us we needed to know everything, and we naively believed it was possible until we had expended our last bits of effort and realized that we would fall short. There was always one more book to read, one more journal article to scan, one more lecture to attend. Total commitment was not enough, and when we embraced that reality, it was humbling, terrifying, frustrating, and liberating all at once.

I never gave up, but I did give in. I gave in to the need to find that diversion that acknowledged my abilities were finite and my patients were mortal even when I did everything I could to relieve suffering or to keep people alive. I looked for flight schools in the Baltimore yellow pages and found three close to home. When I had a weekend off, I visited the schools and asked questions. I met the instructors and took introductory flights. The flight that hooked me occurred on an overcast April afternoon at Glenn L. Martin State airport. Martin had been one of the "Barons of the Sky,"[1] reaping millions selling bombers to the US government before and during World War II. The airport was a monument to his success and had been purchased by the state of Maryland as a general aviation facility and home for the Air National Guard. The old construction hangars made an ideal location for a flight school, and there were several here. The one that captured my attention was sponsored by the Beech Aircraft Company, and they called it the Aero Club. It offered an entire line of aircraft and a complete set of self-taught ground courses to provide preparation for Federal Aviation Administration written tests. The self-instruction format allowed me to learn the material as my residency training allowed.

My demonstration flight on a dreary Sunday afternoon in early April was one of the shortest on record. The ceiling was only 1,200 to 1,500 feet overcast, but I insisted that I have a flight. The proprietor of the flying school, Pete Greene, was very accommodating and loaded me into the left seat of the two-seat Beech Sport trainer. He spoke on the radio to the tower in a curious verbal shorthand, and they must have known that he was escorting a wide-eyed dreamer that gloomy afternoon. We took off on Runway 14, climbed to the base of the clouds, entered the landing pattern with sequential left turns, and landed in less than five minutes. For Pete, it was one part showmanship, one part salesmanship, and a dash of airmanship. For me, it was pure wonder. The world of illness and misery and suffering disappeared in the cockpit of that small craft that Sunday afternoon. I had found the tool that would lead me through many challenging years, providing the very reorientation I needed to regain my perspective so often lost in the rigorous demands of postgraduate medical education.

My first flight with an instructor occurred on April 16, the 290th day of my internship. Sixteen months later, on August 18 of the next year, after patching together training flights during weekends and vacations, I passed my private pilot check ride. During the next decade, I added my commercial certificate and an instrument rating for single-engine aircraft. With the airplane came an opportunity for seeing myself and the world from personal and spiritual heights external to my daily existence in hospitals and clinics, where I was often too close to events to see them clearly. Time and distance shrank when I was at the controls of an aircraft, and somehow, inexplicably, meaning returned to my frenetic life. Medicine, my heart's desire, was a jealous mistress who consumed me without mercy and with no regard for life's competing priorities. Aviation renewed me for myself and, consequently, for my patients.

My introduction to the needs of the sick and dying came in Baltimore years before my internship and my first solo flight. This was where I first learned that true faith drives out fear,[2] and that often we do nothing to aid those who suffer because we fear that what we do will be inadequate. This fear immobilizes us and prevents us from performing small deeds that, when done, are received gratefully by those whose lives we touch.

In the summer of 1972, a summer that would become infamous for the Watergate break-in and cover-up, I was between my sophomore and junior years as an undergraduate at the Johns Hopkins University. The first two years challenged me academically, because my high school preparation, although adequate at a small rural high school, was not equal to the superior preparation my Hopkins classmates received at private preparatory and large public high schools. Though I was eligible for the work/study program from the time I matriculated, I chose to concentrate on my studies during my first two years.

During my sophomore year, President Nixon signed the National Cancer Act. Great public hopefulness for future therapeutic successes followed broad coverage in the national press. I entered college thinking I was going to be a surgeon, championing pioneers like the Mayo brothers and Christiaan Barnard, the heart surgeon, but cancer biology wooed me, and clinical cancer research appeared to offer ever-expanding opportunities. *Why not join the excitement?* I asked myself.

A spectacular chance came to me by fortunate coincidence. At the southern end of the Johns Hopkins Homewood campus was the Wyman Park US Public Health Service Hospital, where Drs. Michael Walker, Nicholas Bachur, and Peter Wiernik directed a basic and clinical research program supported by the National Cancer Institute with increased funding from the National Cancer Act. The program trained the first generation of physicians in the new specialty of medical oncology. The trainees and their faculty offered numerous opportunities for us undergraduates to participate in countless research activities related to cancer.

My first task there, because I did not yet have clinical training, was to collect information about the hospitalized patients, add it to a computer database, and print a daily census report for the staff to use on ward rounds. As I collected data from both the medical records and the physicians, I naturally became more curious about the patients who came from all parts of the United States to the research center because it offered one final glimmer of hope in their battles against diseases that few physicians knew how to treat effectively in 1972. Most patients had lymphatic malignancies and had been referred for treatment with new drugs that showed great promise against this group of cancers. Many patients were young and had traversed the continent to participate in the experimental treatment programs.

As I became more familiar with the routines of the institution and more comfortable with the emotional trauma of seeing patients without hair who were bleeding and infected with virulent bacteria, my mentors allowed me to learn the simple task of drawing blood from the patients. Because we were using new anti-cancer drugs for the first time in humans, we had little understanding about how these chemical toxins might affect bone marrow, liver, and kidney function. We decided to monitor as many hematological and biochemical parameters as we could, once or twice a day, to learn more about the toxicities of the therapies. It was in this setting that I first saw hemorrhagic cystitis (bleeding in the urinary bladder from irritation caused by chemotherapy), cardiomyopathy (weakening of the heart muscle from Adriamycin chemotherapy), and nerve toxicity from vinca alkaloid chemotherapy such as vincristine.

Although we had only thirty-five patients in the research unit, drawing blood was time consuming. The clinicians needed test results by midday so they could make decisions about additional therapy or supportive care. The college students were the ideal task force to collect the morning blood, but I was surprised that the staff permitted me, with my minimal training in the use of a needle and syringe, to perform venipuncture on unsuspecting patients who were unaware that I was such a novice.

Drawing the blood was a challenge because the patients had repeated venipunctures that gradually eliminated the optimal drawing sites. The constant assault with toxic chemotherapy also scarred their veins, necessitating that we use small scalp vein needles inserted into tiny veins on the backs of hands to obtain the twenty or thirty milliliters of blood required each day. The whole procedure each day required a rather prolonged and intimate inspection of the upper extremities of each patient, followed by the most gentle and careful insertion of the small-gauge needle, along with an equally slow and careful withdrawal of the required blood.

This sort of physical intimacy with a seriously ill person was, at first, quite unsettling to me as a technically oriented student venipuncturist. I was asking strangers to allow me, a young college student, to enter the privacy of their illnesses to withdraw a part of them with my unskilled hands that trembled occasionally at the wonder and mystery of it all. As long as I did not consider too seriously what I was doing or to whom I was doing it, I was fine. Relentlessly, though, my anxiety percolated through my flushed skin, and my disquietude, coupled with the intimacy of the touching and probing, forced me to chatter incessantly. It seemed impossible to enter a room every day and not inquire about the patient's home and family, their job, and their favorite recreation.

Bob was a printer from Indianapolis with an aggressive lymphoma that did not respond well to therapy. Early in the long summer of 1972, he looked hopeful and relatively healthy, considering the severity of his illness, but as the weeks passed, the disease and the therapy changed Bob dramatically. He became thin and weak and was confined to bed. As I drew his blood every day, I learned that he had a large printing business that was quite successful. He delighted in hearing about methods used to print our daily census report using a time-sharing computer attached through an acoustic coupler to a teletype printer that used school-grade yellow paper on large rolls, the type Bill Cosby described comically as having large chunks of wood floating in it. Bob and I knew that computers would change profoundly his profession and mine, and we enjoyed speculating about the effects being engendered by the emerging technology. Bob's wife, Karen, enjoyed our conversations, and after a few weeks, I liked both of them a great deal.

Despite the efforts of his physicians, Bob did not get better, and by late July he was dying. As the medical team made rounds each day, it became clear to me that his doctors could offer less and less additional chemotherapy to treat Bob's cancer. The discussions among the team members became briefer with each subsequent visit to his room until the team stopped entering the room at all, talking instead in muted whispers outside his door, his wife anxiously trying to overhear any possibly hopeful news. Our avoidance of the Millers bothered me and struck me as abandonment. (I would not understand this phenomenon fully until fifteen years later when, as the attending physician in charge of a teaching service with ten students and residents, I moved the team quickly past the rooms of dying patients so that we could spend more time with stable, healthier individuals in our care. I visited with families of the dying patients after we completed our work rounds.)

I forced myself to visit Bob's room daily even after the team withdrew orders for blood drawing. It was impossible for me to just stop seeing this new friend who was departing as quickly as he had entered my young life. Yet I was terribly uneasy when I entered his room, because I had nothing to do. I could temporarily ignore his physical infirmities when I drew his blood, but it was far more challenging to look past his wasted temples and extremities, his bruised skin and his dry lips, when I made social visits. The visits became too difficult for both of us, and I became guilty and ashamed of both my revulsion at his demise and my curiosity and fascination with his dying.

How could this be intriguing? But it was, while, at the same time, it was excruciatingly painful because I liked Bob and felt so utterly helpless.

Guilt. Sadness. Curiosity. Helplessness.

For the first time, I was seeing and feeling the emotions of death, and I was very confused. What was I to do for Bob? I didn't know, but I kept visiting. We shared idle chatter, nervous questions, as if we were meeting again for the first time. It made me uncomfortable, but Bob and Karen did not seem to mind.

Then, one afternoon I entered the room as Bob was clearly breathing his last breaths. His respirations were agonal, he was restless, and his wife was distressed. I have never before or since felt so utterly helpless. So I just stood at the side of the bed, stood and watched as his last minutes of life ebbed painfully away. I was frozen, I couldn't move, and I desperately wanted either to leave or to make the whole scene disappear.

Finally, after a long, onerous watch, Karen said, "Would you please get the priest?"

On that day we had exchanged no words before then. We had merely stood in the darkening silence broken only by Bob's labored breathing. I muttered, "Sure" or something equally brief and exited speedily from the room.

Sweet relief! What release! But what to do for Bob? I grabbed the first nurse I could find and pleaded urgently, "Mr. Miller needs a priest!"

The passive and uninspired "All right" from the nurse startled me. *Why am I so concerned if she's not?* I asked myself. *Why is she so calm? Is it her experience? Does she not know my friend Bob? What do I do now? Do I go back into the room?* No one was there to tell me, and I surely did not know. I busied myself with paperwork at the computer table in the nurses' station until the nurse returned to say that Bob had died.

I wanted to return to the room, but I just could not. It was too painful, and I felt terribly inadequate. I was frustrated for days afterward and cursed myself for being so young, so naive and so inexperienced.

Weeks later a letter arrived from Mrs. Miller. I thought it was a bit curious that she should write to me, the most junior person on the entire team. Her letter was warm and personal, and she spoke fondly of the entire medical team who had cared for Bob. She explained that both she and Bob were aware of the seriousness of his illness long before he died. They were grateful for the staff of the cancer center for making an attempt at treatment when others said there was nothing that could be done:

July 31, 1972

Dear Vic,
    Just a few words to thank you for your kindness to the Millers since you came to the B.C.R.C. [Baltimore Cancer Research Center]

Bob and I have both enjoyed getting to know you and talking with you about your work. He always had a great sense of humor, and you didn't seem to mind a little kidding about drawing blood, etc.

We both discussed you and felt you have the making of a fine young doctor. We decided you will have good rapport with your patients because of your fine warm personality.

I especially want to thank you for your kindness to me during Bob's last hours. It really meant a lot.

My best wishes for your future success in the medical profession, and may God bless you in your endeavors.

Sincerely,
Karen Miller
(Mrs. Bob Miller)

Why was she grateful? What had I done? I felt I had failed miserably when a friend needed me. All I had done was to go tell a nurse that the wife of a dying man wanted him to see a priest. What did that mean? Any schoolboy could have carried that message. But I *was* a schoolboy, nothing more. Yes, a twenty-year-old schoolboy, but as much as I wanted to be a physician the day Bob died, as much as I wanted to have magical powers to save him from his ordeal, I would learn years later that even the most gifted physician could not have saved Bob that summer afternoon. That was a lesson I would learn again and again as I encountered the limits of my profession and its inability to save the terminally ill.

She thanked me. Like the astonished Quasimodo who marveled, "She gave me water!" I could not comprehend why Mrs.

Miller thanked me. Why did she do that? After much reflection, I came to understand that it was because, in my simple presence, I had met a need, I had filled a void. This gift required no technical sophistication, no advanced degree, no special training. I merely needed to be available. I have grown to treasure this experience as one of the most valued learning opportunities of my life.

My repeated encounters with the dying ultimately taught me a profound lesson: they do not want magic. They do not need or want eloquent pronouncements. They certainly do not need bedside sermons. They yearn, instead, for the abiding presence of a steady hand, a familiar friend, a calming voice. Theirs is a solo flight more lonely than that of the aerial pioneers. They are pushing the boundaries to points where no one has ever before gone and from which no one has returned, except one. The abiding presence of the friend or family member at the bedside throughout that last perilous journey is as reassuring as the airport beacon at night or the voice of the air traffic controller who guides the aviator safely to his destination.

The loving presence of a friend at the side of one who is dying is an enduring gift not only to the recipient but to the giver. Years later, as I reflected on that afternoon, my feelings of inadequacy and disappointment gave way to the profound sense that I had comforted a friend, that I had helped him navigate safely to the other side.

---

1   Biddle, W. *Barons of the Sky—From Early Flight to Strategic Warfare, the Story of the American Aerospace Industry.* New York: Simon & Schuster, 1991.
2   1 John 4:18.

3

Can You Save Him, Doc?

> I fear no foe, with Thee at hand to bless: Ills have no weight and tears no bitterness. Where is death's sting? Where, grave, thy victory? I triumph still, if Thou abide with me.[1]
>
> —Henry Francis Lyte

Our training as medical residents exposes us to the realities of death and dying, but the ultimate responsibility for those who died while in our care during our internships and residencies remained with our attending physicians who supervised us in our teaching hospitals. When we completed our training, we moved on to new positions where we ourselves became attending physicians. We were now, as licensed physicians for the first time in our careers, solely responsible for the critically ill and dying patients who were under our care. These early experiences further shaped my personal understanding of the meaning of suffering and death. These encounters with death early in my career forced me to wrestle with my own disquieting feelings and with the raw emotions of my patients and their families through what was often cumbersome trial and error. My first exposure to these often unsettling learning experiences occurred while I was an attending physician and a commissioned officer in the United States Public Health Service.

Summersville is the home of the Nicholas County courthouse and some 3,500 inhabitants nestled in the hills of central West Virginia on the Gauley River. The region abounds in the natural beauty of the Appalachians, and the native people are rugged individualists who are fiercely proud of their traditions. They are humble folk, initially suspicious of outsiders and loyal to those who share their bond to the land and its long, proud history.

Proud, loyal individuals strive to provide for their own needs, including health care, even when circumstances, environment, and politics do not foster easy solutions. For years, the residents of Summersville had traveled miles when they required hospitalization while local physicians provided competent outpatient care. Richwood, twenty-two miles east on a winding and scenic road, had a hundred-bed hospital that seldom reached 50 percent occupancy rates. More complete inpatient diagnostic and therapeutic services were available in Beckley, fifty miles to the south, where there were both private and Veterans Administration hospitals. State-of-the-art tertiary care was offered 90 miles away in Charleston or 120 miles north at the University of West Virginia Medical Center in Morgantown.

In the 1960s, before the completion of the interstate highway system, the immediate need for both Summersville and Nicholas County was nursing-home beds. Economics and geography made it infeasible to consider chronic care for the elderly at great distances from home, but the passage of both the Hill-Burton Act and Medicare legislation enabled Summersville to build a chronic-care nursing facility in 1966 with construction funds from state, county, and federal sources.

With the opening of the nursing facility, there arose the possibility that the physicians who cared for the resident elderly population could also provide acute care to the populations of Summersville and Nicholas County. In 1977 one of the nursing care wings was converted to an acute-care facility. An emergency room, operating room, delivery room, and radiology suite were added to or remodeled in the existing structure.

The hospital board recruited a surgeon to augment the small and capable cadre of family physicians practicing in the facility. As the patient volume increased and the community became more confident in the capabilities of the institution, the community demanded diversity of medical expertise: pediatricians, an internist, and an obstetrician/gynecologist. The dilemma for a small town in the 1970s, as it remains now, was how to recruit and retain medical specialists during practice start-up years when patient volume is low and patients gradually learn that the new physician has arrived, that he or she is competent and personable, and that it is no longer necessary to travel fifty or ninety miles or more to obtain medical care. An experimental answer to this problem was proposed in a program of the US Public Health Service known as the National Health Service Corps (NHSC).

The motive behind NHSC was simple: find young physicians in training and recruit them early in their careers to rural, primary-care practices. Attract them by offering medical school stipends and scholarships to relieve the financial burden of a medical education, and extract, in return, an equal number of years of service in needy rural communities. To facilitate the transition from training to practice, NHSC provided salary support to the physician to relieve the financial woes of a fledgling practice, and the community used the practice income to support hiring nursing and clerical personnel.

It was a thoughtful plan, a plan that worked well as an interim solution during the late 1970s and the 1980s. Then, however, the realities and hardships of solo rural practice began to erode the Corps, and physician after physician left to pursue other, less demanding professional pursuits. The Corps proved to be an interesting experiment. A survey of physicians who moved into rural areas between 1987 and 1990 showed that although 51 percent initially anticipated working in underserved areas longer than ten years, only 14 percent expected to remain more than five years in their assigned practices. Three quarters of the physicians felt there were few acceptable practice sites available to them, one-third said they would have preferred urban sites, and two-thirds were matched in states where they had not lived or trained. Corps physicians felt their spouses' and children's needs were less well satisfied in their communities than non-Corps physicians, and Corps physicians reported lower satisfaction in their work and personal lives. Only one-third began serving their communities with intentions to live in the underserved area after their obligations ended. In reporting this study, researchers said the needs and preferences of physicians placed in rural areas were not well met, and low morale and poor retention rates were endemic among Corps physicians.[2]

The imminent and yet unforeseen problems of the NHSC notwithstanding, my fiancée, Sally, and I were confronted with the obstacle of finding continued funding for our medical educations after we met in medical school. Sally was certain that her family would not agree to finance her education after she married; I was already paying for my education, having come from a parsonage of limited means. We were blinded by love but certain that a solution would be forthcoming if we were both patient and persistent. During our second year of medical school, the answer arrived in the NHSC scholarship program. We were fortunate that Sally grew up in a rural community in western Pennsylvania and that I had lived in the Appalachian highlands in the southwestern corner of the state for three years during one of my father's rural pastorates. Our residence histories, and the fact that Sally intended to practice pediatrics and I, internal medicine, made us a natural choice for the Corps. The program even agreed to defer our two-year service commitment until the completion of our residencies three years after graduation from medical school.

In the United States the entire clinical medicine environment changes on the first day of July each year as training programs end and physicians arrive both eager and anxious to begin their new assignments. In keeping with this proud and venerated tradition, Sally and I arrived in Summersville on July 2, delighted to have completed our arduous years of residency training but fearful that we might not be capable of solo practice away from the sheltering cocoon of the academic medical teaching center. We hoped we had learned enough, but we knew we could not possibly have learned all that we needed to know. We wondered if some deficit in knowledge, some careless oversight, or some unintentional omission might result in an adverse outcome for a patient entrusted to our care. We wanted to test our clinical knowledge and prove to ourselves and our new community that we had learned well, yet there was a part of us that hoped no one, not one patient, would enter the clinic door to test our unproven expertise.

Our first ten days were very quiet. We each saw only five or ten patients each day, and no one was ill. Colds, allergies, and poison ivy filled the office schedule. It was the sort of brooding peace known by armies as they face each other in the trenches, guns poised, yet firing no shots.

Our telephone shattered the peace on the second Friday night in our new home on a quiet street a mile from the hospital. The caller was our very talented Korean surgeon, W. Don Joo, who told me he wanted me to see a patient for him.

"I am at the emergency room with Bob Fredrickson," Don told me. "He is a member of our church, and I think he is having a heart attack."

For some reason, probably because of my own anxiety, I did not understand that Don wanted me there *immediately*. The patient, unknown to me at the time of the telephone call, was dying from a massive heart attack that had destroyed most of his cardiac septum, the wall in the heart that separates the two main pumping chambers.

"You want me to see him now?" I asked.

"You better come right away," Don replied.

My blood ran cold. This was a trip I did not want to make. Memories of the halcyon days of my recently completed internship filled my troubled mind, days when the emergency room would call to offer me the mandatory "privilege" of accepting a dying man to my keeping in the coronary care unit in the wee hours of the morning.

∞

Imagine a family sitting quietly at home watching television, reading the newspaper, involved with hobbies. Suddenly, with no warning, their father is stricken with severe, agonizing chest pain. He has had a history of angina pectoris (heart-related chest pain), and is under a doctor's care. Now, though, he is in such intense pain that he cannot speak. His face begins to turn blue as he clutches at his chest. Family members, horrified and confused, attempt to administer nitroglycerine under his tongue, but it provides no relief.

Realizing the severity of the situation, the man's son calls the local city ambulance through the 911 network. Before the ambulance arrives three minutes later, the man stops breathing, and after a few bewildering seconds, one of the man's daughters begins cardiopulmonary resuscitation. Other family members watch in anguished silence, struggling simultaneously with feelings of shock, helplessness, fear, and indescribable apprehension.

After only minutes that feel like eternity, the ambulance crew bursts into the family living room with as much care and respect as is possible under the circumstances but largely ignoring the family and focusing fully on the man lying on the floor being resuscitated by his daughter. They move her aside, not having time or inclination to thank her. She steps back a few feet, stands for a moment in silent disbelief, and then runs crying to the next room as stunned, nearly numb, family members follow. A few remain in the living room, not really wishing to observe the resuscitation, but unsure just where they should be or what they should do.

After a fifteen-minute attempt to revive the victim, he regains a pulse but not consciousness. During the resuscitation, the patient has vomited on the living room floor, on himself, and on some of the participants. While inserting intravenous lines to administer drugs into the patient's arms, the ambulance crew allows several ounces of blood to drip onto the floor. Periodically, the family members standing in the adjacent room peer into the living room, terrified and unsure what is happening. Neighbors are summoned by the family. Those not called soon arrive out of curiosity to inspect the scene, attracted by the steady flashing of the ambulance's red and white lights. Outside the home on a narrow residential city street, a crowd of onlookers gathers.

After twenty minutes, the ambulance crew is ready to remove the tenuously stable patient to the waiting ambulance. The family, finally certain that their loved one has not yet succumbed, but consumed with fear, try to decide what to do next. Helpful neighbors organize a hasty carpool to the hospital. Great confusion surrounds the seemingly simple arrangements, and family members begin to identify necessary but uncompleted tasks as they crowd into waiting vehicles. Neighbors assure the family that the house will be watched, absent family members will be called and advised, and latecomers will be directed to the hospital. Their pastor is summoned to the hospital.

Back in the 1980s in the emergency room of the city hospital, a radiotelephone box beeped loudly enough to be heard above the din of the evening's activities. The call was answered by a nurse who recorded the patient's vital signs read by the paramedic in the ambulance, now just three minutes from the hospital. The nurse summoned the emergency room resident, already busy with six patients in various states of distress. The patient in the ambulance, he is told, is unresponsive to physical stimuli but has a systolic blood pressure of 90 millimeters of mercury and an irregular, thready pulse of 110 per minute. He is intubated with an esophageal obturator airway, and the crew is breathing for him with an Ambu bag at a rate of twenty breaths per minute with 50 percent oxygen. They report that the cardiac monitor in their ambulance shows a supraventricular tachycardia with frequent ventricular extrasystoles (a rapid heart rate with lots of extra beats). Using the same technology that NASA used to send heartbeat information back to Earth from manned space flights, the ambulance crew beams an electrocardiogram rhythm strip to the waiting physician. The resident suggests that lidocaine be administered to control the heart rate and rhythm, and the crew complies. The entire interaction takes ninety seconds, and the crew advises they will be at the emergency room door in two minutes.

The resident hangs up the phone and begins to round up support. "Case coming to the major room!" he barks at the intern.

The harried intern makes feeble excuses to explain his rapid departure to a middle-aged woman who has waited three hours to be seen for back pain. She will have to wait another hour for the intern to return.

The medical resident continues to summon assistance: the surgical resident is asked to stand by to place a long intravenous line into the patient's subclavian vein; the respiratory therapy technician is asked to make ready a ventilator for the intubated patient; the overworked radiology technician is advised that a STAT (immediate) portable chest X-ray will be needed within fifteen minutes. The anesthesia resident is paged to the emergency room by the hospital operator, whose usual monotonous tones are raised with a feverish sense of urgency:

"Anesthesia STAT to the emergency room! Anesthesia STAT to the emergency room!"

Throughout the hospital, residents, interns, and support personnel drop their tasks and literally jog to the ER. Bewildered hospital visitors watch white-coated house staff streak by en route to the crisis.

In the major room of the emergency department, all is in readiness. Nurses and physicians pace nervously as they await the arrival of the ambulance. The resident gives last-minute instructions to the visibly anxious intern, who, silently and to himself, tries to no avail to remember at least one thing to do in such a situation. He comforts himself by deciding to do whatever the resident tells him to do. The near-breathless anesthesia resident arrives on the scene, somewhat irritated when he finds he has gotten there ahead of the patient. On a table to the side of the waiting litter are placed the instruments and apparatus necessary for the impending arrival. The respiratory therapist wheels in a ventilator and attaches the oxygen supply from the wall outlet. The head nurse plugs in a cardiac monitor next to the litter and attaches three chest leads to the waiting machine. A half-dozen intravenous bottles hang from ceiling hooks surrounding the litter, their coiled plastic tubing reaching to, but not yet touching, the clean litter sheet. This is the last ordered moment to be seen in this room for the next hour and a half.

Just as the intern asks, "Where are they?" the ambulance crew arrives with the patient on a wheeled stretcher. The patient's soiled shirt is torn open, and plastic cardiac lead patches are stuck to his reddened skin. Telltale circular burns mark the skin where defibrillator paddles have been applied and discharged. There is a reeking odor of vomit and blood and sweat. The ambulance crew looks both fatigued and relieved to be at their destination. A great scurrying about immediately ensues as nurses, physicians, and technicians individually and collectively do their separate and vital tasks. The anesthesia resident removes the esophageal obturator and deftly inserts an endotracheal tube. The ventilator is turned on, and its rhythmic, cycling cadence quietly directs the proceedings, acting as a sort of medical metronome. The intern places a nasogastric tube, and the resident obtains a sample of arterial blood. Nurses attach IV tubing to plastic venous catheters already in the patient's arm veins. An electrocardiogram is recorded. The resident observes that it is diagnostic of an acute anterior myocardial infarction (i.e., a heart attack). Venous blood is drawn and sent to the laboratory for a score of diagnostic tests.

The nurse in charge of the shift reminds the resident that no one has spoken to the family members who are huddled in the waiting room that is too small to accommodate all of them comfortably. The resident is reluctant to face yet another group of anxious strangers for whom he has only incomplete answers.

"Yes, your father is alive. Yes, he is critically ill. Yes, we believe he has suffered a serious heart attack. He will be in the cardiac care unit for days, more than a week if he survives."

The scene is tense with strangers sharing intimacies they would never offer in other circumstances. The family wants to trust this stranger, this necessary intruder into their lives, because he holds so much in his hands, he and many other strangers they have not yet met and many they will never meet. Some of the strangers they will wish never to have known because they bear such unwelcome news.

The door to the emergency room swings open. A team of four is wheeling the patient to the elevator. The family stares in silent, motionless disbelief. Women sob as men gaze downward, too numb to be angry, too unpracticed to cry.

The resident excuses himself from the emotional scene, hoping to avoid being a voyeur to others' grief, offering the excuse that there are other patients who need him. He backs away slowly while reciting sympathies that are more objective and intellectual than passionate, yet real nonetheless. The family moves in their collectively stunned uneasiness toward the elevator at the end of the hall, wondering silently how this happened and what additional pain and suffering lurk in their suddenly uncertain and fearsome futures.

⁂

But my situation in rural West Virginia on this July evening was different. There wasn't a cardiologist within fifty miles. I was it, the last line of defense, and I was about to make decisions about the care of this man without the benefit of consultations, without sophisticated monitoring, aided by nurses and a physician whom I hardly knew. This was not good, and I was anxious about the coming hours for both my patient and myself. Why had I not thought of this before? All physicians in training know that the day will come when they will be examined not on paper in the endless written evaluations we faced repeatedly, but in real life, with real patients.

My first solo flight as an attending physician had arrived unplanned and unscheduled.

How can you be scared, Vogel? I chastised myself. *If you go to the hospital showing anything other than total self-control, no one in this town is going to trust anything you do for the next two years! You have been trained for this. Do what you can and get on with it!*

Having completed the mini-sermon to myself, I told Sally where I was going, slid into the car, and arrived at the hospital in five minutes.

What I found was more terrifying than any of the vivid fantasies I had visualized in my car during the dark and brief drive to the hospital. Mr. Fredrickson was sitting fully upright in the bed closest to the door in the tiny two-bed coronary-care unit. All of the lights were on (unusual for this time of the night), and two very worried nurses hovered around the bed. Dr. Joo was talking quietly to the patient, who was ashen gray. A re-breathing oxygen mask hung on his face, and he intermittently opened and closed his eyes as he gasped in short, shallow breaths.

"Cardiogenic shock," I muttered to myself. We were in deep trouble. It meant that the damage to his heart muscle was so extensive that he could not sustain normal blood pressure. I was fearful that his death was imminent.

I hurriedly introduced myself to both the nurses and Mr. Fredrickson. I was certain he had no idea who I was, nor would he, even if his now poorly perfused brain were working normally. I wasn't even sure that the nursing staff knew me, because this was my first patient in the hospital.

Don Joo and the nurses quickly recounted the unfortunate history of Bob Fredrickson. He had been at home with his family when he experienced chest pain while playing cards. He became nauseated and slumped in his chair. His family wanted to take him to his doctor in Charleston, ninety miles away. Mr. Fredrickson told them it was too far to go and that he wanted to go to Summersville Memorial Hospital at once. On arrival, his electrocardiogram showed the classic findings of an extensive heart attack involving virtually all twelve leads of his EKG tracing. His blood pressure was low, his pulse thready and rapid, his skin cold and clammy. He was in shock because his damaged heart simply could not pump blood with any efficiency. He was dying in front of us.

Before my arrival, the team had administered lidocaine intravenously because Mr. Fredrickson's cardiac rhythm was irregular, and despite beginning a dopamine infusion to elevate his falling blood pressure, it remained low. The damage to his heart was extensive and irreparable, and the clinical situation was becoming hopeless.

I wanted to run, to be anywhere but there. We were out of options, and my only comfort was my training and experience that told me that there would be little to do even if we were at one of the academic, tertiary referral hospitals in which I had trained. Pacemakers, thrombolytic therapy, and invasive digital pressure monitoring were all incapable of saving a heart that had been as extensively damaged as Bob Fredrickson's was.

As much as I tried to concentrate on caring for my patient, thoughts about my failing reputation kept intruding. All I could imagine was how my future for the next two years would be adversely affected by the death of my first hospitalized patient in this rural outpost.

In the hall outside the CCU, Mr. Fredrickson's family had assembled during the half hour we had been attending to him. They were literally huddled in a circle with their pastor, and it was clear to me that they grasped the severity of the situation. I reluctantly intervened when it appeared they had concluded their prayer. I explained who I was and that I had been called in by Dr. Joo because of my training and experience in internal medicine. (As my years in Summersville progressed, I began to understand that few people know what internal medicine is. One patient offered, "Oh yeah, I know what that is. You're one of them rookie doctors!" No sir, not an intern, I explained. I am an internist. He returned an empty stare.)

The family was not impressed, either. "We want him to go to Charleston," said one of the older sons. I explained that an hour ride in an ambulance now would be at least ill advised and at worst, fatal. I further suggested that they could do little at the hospital and persuaded them, with some effort, to go home.

In retrospect, that recommendation was a mistake. After the family left, Mr. Fredrickson's clinical situation deteriorated progressively. Within a half hour, he sustained a full cardiac arrest. Dr. Joo and I resuscitated him for twenty minutes, but the situation was hopeless. His heart had been destroyed by the lack of blood and oxygen as a result of the heart attack.

Now I faced the terrible task of calling the family and breaking the news. I employed the spineless dodge often used by physicians in dire clinical circumstances. I asked the nurse to call and say the situation was grave. This would save me the embarrassment of having to answer questions on the phone, or worse, having to lie.

The family arrived with their pastor within ten minutes. The looks on their faces told me that they knew what I would be telling them before I spoke a word.

"Mr. Fredrickson died," I said. "I am very sorry. The damage to his heart was so extensive that nothing could save him. He would have died on the way to Charleston," I assured them. They just nodded. I was sure they thought my inadequacies had killed their loved one.

The weekend that followed was not a good one, and the next week was not much better because my racing thoughts would not be quieted. I was certain that word was out all over town that the new, young doctor had failed his first test. I was sure I was professionally ruined in Nicholas County, even though my rational self told me I had done absolutely nothing wrong. My horror intensified when the Nicholas *Chronicle*, the local weekly newspaper, had a picture of my patient on the front page of its next issue, exactly one week after the tragic event. Mercifully, they did not mention my name in the accompanying article.

As the months passed, I learned how foolish all my fears had been. After trying another congregation, Sally and I joined Mr. Fredrickson's church, where his wife was the organist. We got to know the family quite well, visited their home on several occasions, and saw them frequently at social functions. They did not hold me responsible for Bob's death. Instead, they thanked me for being willing to try to save him. They even saw the dark irony in my having sent them home from the hospital just before Bob died, and they understood my motives when I explained that he might have lived for hours.

It is a lonely, frightful duty to tell a family their loved one has died after you have reached the limits of your knowledge and skills. When you have done all you know how to do, nothing remains but to admit your constraints and face the sadness of life's finitude. I never feel so hollow, so inadequate, though, as when I know there is nothing more to do medically for a patient. It is a worse feeling in many ways than realizing you have overlooked or forgotten something, because the latter is one man's failing, a fact that can be faced, accepted, and corrected. The former is the admission of our collective ignorance, with consequences far more grave.

---

1. Lyte, Henry Francis. "Abide with Me," 1847 ("Eventide") Wm. H. Monk, 1861. (#51, The Hymnal of the Evangelical and Reformed Church, St. Louis, 1941).
2. Pathman DE et al. The National Health Service Corps experience for rural physicians in the late 1980s. *JAMA* 1994;272:1341–1348.

4

Understanding Suffering Through Reason

> How miserable it is to have to stand in mute sorrow with nothing to say to those we love, when they are in great pain.[1]
> —Thomas Merton

As I struggled to understand my own response to suffering, I began by looking at the responses of those I saw around me. It seemed to me in my distress that the most important question was "Why is it reasonable that a loving God should allow us to suffer and die?" As a Christian, I felt compelled to explain suffering and death because the relief of suffering is the central meaning of the healing miracles of Jesus Christ, and his incarnation, passion, and resurrection are the defining events of the gospels. My difficulty with a God who would allow us to suffer and die arises from the culturally acquired assumptions I was taught as a member of our materialistic society. We believe that pleasure, particularly physical pleasure, is the highest good. Having embraced that moral position, any consideration of the meaning and value of suffering becomes intellectually untenable. As a society, we appear to derive our "salvation" from materialistic, technological solutions. To suppose that salvation (Latin *salvus*, that is, health) could derive from a beneficent, loving God becomes anathema because God seems invisible and uncaring. And that was the question I would ask after several years of practice during my mother's death: "Where are you, God, as my beloved mother is dying?"[2]

Very early in my academic career, I served as chairman of a breast cancer panel at the American Cancer Society's Science Writers Seminar in San Diego. My role was to guide the national press through a briefing designed to explain in lay language the scientific abstracts the reporters were about to hear. After the session, one of the molecular geneticists and I took a cab ride to Sea World nearby. As I watched the trained dolphins, sea lions, and killer whales perform their trained acts, I was reminded of the command in Genesis for humankind to have dominion over the animals. Then, as I walked through the marine aquarium and viewed the moon jellyfish, spiny crabs, tiny shrimp, anemones, and the countless creatures of creation, I was reminded that we are created, as are the animals. We are here by design, not by accident. I gazed in wonder at the nautilus and thought of Lewis Thomas's book *The Medusa and the Snail*.[3] It is brilliant prose that actually evoked my own personal theology. I believe that we are not an accident of the random couplings of organic molecules. How ironic that earlier in the day I had spoken of DNA restriction mapping to the science writers. DNA is the stenographer's transcript of the designer's (i.e., God's) blueprint, a blueprint that permits the evolution of biological diversity.

I realized that I was being impeded in my understanding of suffering by my materialism that indulged the evolutionists and affirmed that we are here by accident, through some cataclysm in the primordial soup that randomly allowed atoms to coalesce into proteins, and proteins, in turn, to synthesize larger molecules that would subsequently direct the synthesis of new proteins.[4] This was the scientific training in which I was instructed, but the sheer mathematical odds against the improbable series of evolutionary events arrested my materialist leanings. For me, there was a fallacy in this logic because our being here is so statistically improbable. We have not had an infinite amount of time to let creation occur, so I struggled and wrestled with answers that science provided but that could not satisfy my personal longing for a more complete resolution to my own questions about suffering.

Dr. Francis Collins, medical geneticist, former head of the Human Genome Project, and now director of the National Institutes of Health, refers to what he calls "theistic evolution" and says that this belief has six premises: (1) the physical universe came into being out of nothingness about 14 billion years ago; (2) the properties of the universe appear to have been precisely tuned for life despite huge improbabilities; (3) once life arose, the processes of evolution and natural selection permitted the development of biological diversity and complexity; (4) once evolution got under way, no special supernatural intervention was required; (5) humans are part of this process, sharing a common ancestor with the great apes; and (6) humans are unique in ways that defy evolutionary explanation and point to our spiritual nature.[5] Dr. Collins says, "God intentionally chose [the elegant mechanism of evolution] to give rise to special creatures who would have intelligence, a knowledge of right and wrong, free will, and a desire to seek fellowship with him."[6]

I am not a literal Biblical creationist, and I certainly do not believe that the world is only some 4,000 or 5,000 years old, but I have enough statistical ability and comprehension to know that nothing so complicated as human life could have evolved by accident in even the relatively long period of time that life has been on this planet. More important, the implications of my believing that life arose as an accident are grimly serious. If I consider, for example, a child who learns that his birth was unplanned, that he was the product of an accidental conception, I can anticipate that that child likely will feel, at least at times, unwanted and unaccepted and will view his environment as hostile and unforgiving. If I try to believe that human life is here as a result of chance, I must conceptualize a hostile world where my continued existence is as improbable as my initial appearance. For me, acceptance of a random, evolutionary theory precludes the possibility that a loving, caring God could exist and makes it nearly, if not absolutely, impossible that such a God could intervene personally in my suffering.

There are roughly 3 *billion* total base pairs in the human genome,[7] with only four distinct base pairs, but if I accept that these compounds (which are, themselves, relatively complex molecules having unique and specific structures) coalesced at random through the evolutionary process in the unique and defining arrangement that codes for a human being, I am forced to grapple with the staggering reality that this event had a likelihood of 1 in 4 raised to the 3 billionth power of ever occurring by chance. This, in turn, is equal to 10 raised to the 2.4 billionth power, a number that exceeds the dimensions of the celestial universe!

It is simply impossible for me to argue the origin of human life as a consequence of a series of random events when there has not been enough time since the origin of the universe to permit this spectacular phenomenon to occur by chance. Yet I have been surrounded by knowledgeable, enlightened, scientific minds who make this argument. I cannot accept their view of reality. As I view the evidence, even the origin of a species much simpler than humans is impossible by chance alone because the statistical probability of the random events is astronomically remote.

If I accept creation from randomness alone, then I must conclude that a mechanistic, stochastic view of life evolving by chance suggests that the odds are against us, and that our time is short. The god that I perceive from this worldview is the material god of atoms and chance, a hostile physical force that cannot and does not have the capacity to create us, to know us, or to love us individually. I believe that the pervasive ennui of our present culture is a result of our stark acceptance that we are simply a statistical phenomenon destined to be replaced by the next evolutionary creature in our own inexorable cascade to oblivion. I have sometimes witnessed this fatalism in both my patients and my colleagues. In this mathematical reductionism, they embrace hopelessness, the sentinel emotion of a collective anxiety. Consequently, the extinction of any species troubles some observers greatly and can give rise to a haunting suspicion that our own personal extinction might be the next event in the progressive, programmed flight into nothingness.

With time being short and the odds being against us, there is little to prevent us from self-destruction and ultimate annihilation as we attempt to fulfill the tenets of the materialistic, Darwinian evolution that we have so completely embraced with so little question or examination. If we believe that only the fittest survive, then our lot in life is to determine just how fit we are for the struggle. If we embrace biological determinism, we preclude the possibility of divine providence, and my worldview will come to embody the notion that providence simply cannot intervene in my everyday life. Yet providence is an essential, historical facilitator for my understanding of the very nature of God.[8]

When we perceive self-annihilation—either consciously or unconsciously—to be a likely possibility, our pervasive emotions become, predictably, fear and guilt. Materialistic determinism dictates that my disappearance (and our collective disappearance as a species) is programmed, and it further requires that my very being is derived solely from what I do. The psychological mechanisms whereby we then deal with our guilt are complex, but two prevalent mechanisms that I see in my patients and our culture are compulsive consumption of material goods and sexual promiscuity. For most modern Americans in whom being is doing, the doing is in producing goods and services, and the being is embodied in consuming: "I consume, therefore I am." This, in turn, engenders in us a paradox of compulsive consumption that challenges our own micro- and macro-environments, and we are then forced, in our guilt, to protect vanishing species by restricting our materialist assaults upon the very environment we are simultaneously exploiting and protecting. More disturbing, our consumption is not just of manufactured, physical goods but also of career opportunities, spouses, environmental resources, and social advantages. Sex, interestingly, becomes the mystical religion of our unfulfilled longings.

The Death of God and the Loss of Meaning

When we remove divine providence and substitute a deterministic social equation, our own self-destructive behavior becomes predominant. We then accept physical, educational, social, cultural, or biological events that appear to determine our futures to be demonstrations of our programmed fates in which God cannot and does not participate. But when tragedy supervenes, suffering without God becomes so bleak, so abhorrent, and so terrifying to us that we leave it unaddressed and ignored, both intellectually and emotionally. We refuse to face suffering through willful, direct confrontation. As a consequence, we now believe that the possibility of pleasure being unattainable is so antithetical that pain and suffering have become the ultimate taboo in our culture, which worships deterministically derived physical pleasures. When we reject or deny the reality of pain and suffering, we permit, and perhaps even promote, acceptance of active euthanasia as a proximate but temporary solution to our physical suffering.[9] Avoidance of suffering for us is preferable to confrontation and evaluation, to examination with understanding, when we have excluded God from our experience of pain, grief, and sorrow.

What are the spiritual consequences in our lives when we declare God dead, when we believe events occur at random, when suffering has no meaning? My patients who do so demonstrate a pervading sense of hopelessness and helplessness. These paired emotions give rise to deep frustration that follows a resignation to life that is pointless and void of purpose. If God ignores us so completely that he allows us to suffer and die, then we, like neglected children, must believe that nothing really matters because no one is paying attention. We are not passive by nature, and our frustration over the absence of meaning quickly leads, consequently, to anger that is best characterized as our resentment toward the realities of the creation that is disordered, as we perceive it. This anger leads to violence that we direct toward ourselves and others. The outward manifestations of this anger vary, depending on our unique societal and family environments.

Our pathological preoccupation with violence as the tacit symbol for physical pain on television and in cinema becomes the logical accompaniment of our societal taboo if we insist on evaluating physical suffering only abstractly and at a distance rather than through personal contemplation of the reality of our suffering or the suffering of our loved ones. Contemplation of our own suffering and death ironically becomes too intimate for us to condone when, in fact, our only intimacy is in the search for new physical pleasures. Our avoidance of personal suffering and that of our loved ones then engenders a paradox. As a physician, I have observed that the ultimate intimacy is in my participation in the suffering of others, but that is precisely the intimacy that we actively avoid when we perceive that God is not a full participant in our pain. We exclude him because our view of the world allows no room for him, and then we blame him for being distant and unavailable. Because of our fearfulness and false belief that we have no Advocate or Comforter, we choose to learn less and less about death and about God's design for immortal life. We turn increasingly to graphic portrayals of violence to satisfy our curiosity about death as well as to satiate our physical lusts and our need for vicarious aggression that gives life to our survivalist proclivities.

A more reasoned approach to death is through contemplation, through analysis of calamity, and, most important, through active participation in the death of the saints, those whom we love in our families and in our daily lives. A life of love that is directed specifically toward our fellow human beings must first confront death and personal mortality with the confident assurance of eternal life.

Living without God

When there is no room for the spiritual, or for the possibility of realities existing beyond those that are immediately tangible, we make furtive attempts to capture spiritual realities through a turn to mysticism or other constructs that attempt to connect our physical selves to spiritual realities. We especially embrace those features that direct our focus inwardly where we can be comfortable with our self-absorption and temporarily forget our pain. Ultimately, though, through its distant impersonality and focus on our tangibly physical dimension, mysticism makes itself incapable of providing sufficient explanations for our fallen and suffering world.

When we become too scientific and laden with cultural sophistication, we deny an ancient theological reality that pits the forces of good against those of evil,[10] a pervasive warfare that is more encompassing than any military engagement, either conceived or realized. There is an eternal struggle for control of the earth, wherein one of the forces will win. We might argue that suffering is always a result of the forces of evil overpowering the forces of good, if only temporarily, but we have become too sophisticated to embrace such logic.[11] The recognition of this eternal struggle is, however, the first step in addressing the problem of suffering.

Paradoxically, scientific skeptics have great difficulty with Christianity and its physical, ethical foundation (i.e., its uniquely personal relationship to the living God), but when we allow the reality of this intimacy to suffuse us, our Christian spirituality engenders our concern for both the physical and the infinite. In the ministries of Christ in the Gospels—the miracles of healing and feeding, the resurrection and its celebration—are, for me, the tangible proof and the physical foundation of my faith.[12]

Although the assignment of anthropomorphic qualities to God is fraught with risk, I can be sure that he is utterly consistent in his interactions with human beings. Our faith traditions teach us nothing less. I cannot imagine, for example, that in the person of Jesus Christ at the wedding in Cana, God would have changed water into wine if it were not his intention that people should drink a bit too much and merrily celebrate the marriage of two people from their community. It also appears significant that this miracle occurred at a wedding, which in itself is a mystical combination of our physical and spiritual selves. The message from the first miracle is that we are always both spiritual and physical, and Christianity alone resolves this seemingly incongruent dualism by combining these spiritual manifestations with our true physical reality in a living, historical man who was like us in his own personal suffering and death on our behalf. In our scientific sophistication we are not inclined, however, to embrace miracles. Our penchant, instead, is to search for rational, scientific explanations for observable events. Removing the miraculous is a necessary result of our having removed God as creator and sustainer.

Dr. M. Scott Peck, in his groundbreaking book *The People of the Lie*, showed us that the prevalent human emotion where violence and evil rule the social order is not hate, for hate is not the opposite of love.[13] The opposite of love, according to Peck, is fear, and he provides ample evidence to support the notion that fear, manifested as violence and neglect, is the pervasive emotion in our society. In the upper class, fear leads to unending competition and greed through a persistent pyramid structure that, by design, rewards only the most ruthlessly aggressive. In the middle class, fear causes violence that is maliciously self-destructive. Alcoholism, spousal and child abuse, infidelity, and materialism all have their roots in this fear. Made most visible by the media among the socioeconomically disadvantaged, violence takes its most tangible form in drug abuse, homicide, and prostitution.

No matter what its form, the fuel for our anger-engendered violence is our fears, and the greatest fear among us is not death but rather the fear of isolation and isolated suffering, without friends or loved ones and without God. In the meaningless, random world we have created in our perceptions and fantasies, we are most alone and most fearful. The terrible reality of the outer darkness we have created engenders deep anxieties that come through our separation from the love of God, from those we love and from those who love us; our separation from others is separation from the love of God himself, because he loves us most specifically when he loves us through another person.

From my clinical experience, it appears evident to me that most human suffering is not willfully inflicted by God as punishment. Most suffering, rather, is a result of our obstinate disobedience.[14]

It is not God's intention that we suffer any more than it is my intention as a parent to see my child suffer. Yet, it is on this point that those who profess not to believe in God falter because they simply cannot accept a loving God who allows suffering. We preclude, of course, any possibility that God would intervene in our suffering when we believe he does not exist or that he is unconcerned with human pain. This, though, is the existential reality of modern suffering, because we believe we suffer alone without the possibility of grace. Framed in this context, the problem of our suffering is beyond our own contemplation and frustrates our attempts at rational explanations. As a result, we are left mournfully to our own individual hopelessness.

Faith or Consequences

It is increasingly expensive to replace hope with faith in technology alone, and there are consequences if we attempt to solve our spiritual problems in the physical realm. We all want security and assurances about our futures. We want to avoid pain and suffering, and we want to know that when suffering comes, there will be a quick and comforting solution. Many of my patients seek assurances against suffering in the technology that we have learned to substitute for faith and compassion, and this search, too, has associated costs.

It is clear that physicians, patients, hospitals, employers, and payers are all under a great deal of pressure now to contain health care costs in the United States. Expenditures for health care in 2011 consumed 18 percent of our domestic economic resources, and the appetite of Americans for health care grows continuously.

We will devote 20 percent of our resources to health care in just a few more years.[15] When we are patients, we expect medical technology to repair our ills, and we demand that someone else pay for it. By moving payment for health care resources away from us consumers who generate the expenditures, and by placing the burden on third-party sources, we have removed the usual check on unbridled demand. By placing our faith in the physical, technical sectors of health care, we have fostered demand, even created it where none existed previously. By making medicine a business owned by large corporations that are traded publicly, we have institutionalized rising demand by making it profitable for everyone who shares in our complex system.[16]

Institutionalized demand has profound costs. When I am asked to provide medical oncology consultations for women with newly diagnosed breast cancer, my first concern is to assure that the disease is confined to the breast before we embark on systemic treatments. To assure or, rather, to demonstrate, that the disease is confined at the time of diagnosis, we routinely conduct a battery of tests that include low-technology procedures such as complete blood counts and serum chemistry determinations. These are sometimes supplemented by higher-technology imaging studies such as computerized tomographic (CT) scans of the abdomen to exclude liver metastases, and we occasionally complement these images with PET scans to demonstrated areas of active metastases. We then take the patient to a technologically based primary intervention (i.e., surgery) as the initial treatment for their breast cancer, and after the surgical treatment, there is usually a period of chemotherapy accompanied by more laboratory testing.

Doctor, What if it Were Your Mother?

All of this appears to be very good medicine, and it is, but it imparts to the patient the false belief that technology defines health, and in this we do our patients a disservice. I have been a member of a review committee for my professional society— the American Society of Clinical Oncology (ASCO)— that was charged with examining the evidence regarding what laboratory and imaging studies are appropriate after a woman has completed her therapy for breast cancer. The committee comprised physicians from a number of the country's major university cancer centers and included experts in medical oncology, diagnostic testing, clinical epidemiology, and health economics. Using well-established rules of clinical evidence, the committee reviewed an extensive body of literature concerned with the value of laboratory and radiographic testing after the completion of therapy for breast cancer. The committee met to review the data, discussed the available medical literature, prepared a draft document, discussed it further, and prepared written summaries that were critiqued by peer reviewers both for our society's professional journal and its board of directors.

The final results of that process have been several published documents that recommend no laboratory testing for a woman with breast cancer after her therapy is completed.[17] The committee recommended only physical examinations and annual mammography during the years that follow completion of active therapy. This strategy has been termed "minimalist" by one of the members of the committee who, nevertheless, agreed with the recommendations.

Our statements created an unintended crisis for oncologists and their patients. We are not a nation that is happy with doing nothing or with doing very little. We demand action. We are extremely anxious when we simply wait, and we delude ourselves into thinking that doing something, even if it is not helpful, is better than doing nothing at all. Sometimes, though, doing something merely for the purpose of being active is ultimately detrimental. When our ASCO committee examined the evidence regarding the ability of laboratory testing to identify metastases from breast cancer earlier rather than later, we discovered that testing yielded a number of so-called "false positive" results. That is, if we test healthy women regularly with perfectly acceptable laboratory and imaging procedures, the test results will be abnormal *by chance* some of the time. On further testing, these preliminary abnormal results are found to be normal, and we then conclude that there is actually no recurrence of the breast cancer. Instead of making the situation better, however, the testing makes the situation worse by generating extraordinary and understandable anxiety in the patient about the possibility of recurrent or advanced breast cancer and by creating the need to perform additional testing and added expense. At one level, anxiety among both physicians and patients about disease recurrence is generating health care costs that are not associated with meaningful benefit.

We also discovered, to our surprise, that all this testing actually worsens the quality of the life of a woman with breast cancer—or any other cancer, for that matter—by identifying those patients who do suffer a recurrence of their disease weeks to months before they would have been told their cancer had recurred had we waited for the onset of symptoms or detection of an abnormality on physical examination by their physician. The reason for the decline in the quality of life is that when a patient realizes her cancer has recurred, she understandably becomes profoundly depressed. She realizes that she now faces an uphill struggle against a difficult adversary that she and her physician ultimately cannot defeat. Furthermore, the treatment itself is associated with moderate to severe symptoms that further diminish her well-being and quality of life. Metastatic cancer is a disease that can be controlled but not cured. While there is always hope of a prolonged period of coexistence with metastatic disease, it is much better to have metastases and have no symptoms than to be told the cancer is present in liver or lungs or bones and feel perfectly well. Knowledge of the metastatic disease shatters any sense of hope and safety.

This paradox creates a dilemma for our patients and for us physicians. We constantly admonish patients to obtain regular examinations, not to ignore symptoms, and to seek prompt attention for them. Yet we, a body of professional experts, reached the conclusion that it was better to observe than to search for disease in women with breast cancer who have no symptoms. When I attempt to explain this to my patients, some are truly puzzled. My patients expect me to do laboratory tests. If I don't order them, I appear to be either unknowledgeable or insensitive or both. It is difficult for patients to accept that doing nothing may be best because we physicians have conditioned them to think and do otherwise. It is a natural result of our manner of thinking about health and disease, and it incurs financial, emotional, and spiritual costs.

---

[1] Merton, Thomas. *No Man Is an Island*. New York: Harcourt, Brace Jovanovich, 1983, 86.
[2] Psalm 130:1,2.
[3] Thomas, L. *The Medusa and the Snail: More Notes of a Biology Watcher*. New York: Penguin USA, 1995.
[4] See, for example, Behe, MJ. *Darwin's Black Box*. New York: The Free Press, 1996; Denton, M. *Evolution: A Theory in Crisis*. Bethesda,

MD: Adler & Adler, 1985; Haught JF. *God After Darwin—A Theory of Evolution.* Oxford: Westview Press, 2000; Johnson, PE. *Darwin on Trial*, Washington, DC: Regnery Gateway, 1991; Johnson, PE. *Defeating Darwinism by Opening Minds.* Downers Grove, IL: InterVarsity Press, 1997.

[5] Collins, Francis S. *The Language of God: A Scientist Presents Evidence for Belief.* New York: Free Press, 2006, 200.

[6] Ibid, p. 201.

[7] Medawar, PB. *The Limits of Science.* New York: Harper & Row, 1984. Horgan, J. *The End of Science.* New York: Addison-Wesley, 1996. Schroeder, GL. *The Science of God.* New York: The Free Press, 1997. Glynn, P. *God-The Evidence.* Rocklin, CA: Prima Publishing, 1997.

[8] *The Heidelberg Catechism, 400th Anniversary Edition*, Philadelphia: United Church Press, 1963.

Question 27: What do you understand by the providence of God?

"The almighty and ever-present power of God whereby he still upholds, as it were by his own hand, heaven and earth together with all creatures, and rules in such a way that leaves and grass, rain and drought, fruitful and unfruitful years, food and drink, health and sickness, riches and poverty, and everything else, come to us not by chance but by his fatherly hand." (p. 32)

Question 28: What advantage comes from acknowledging God's Creation and providence?

"We learn that we are to be patient in adversity, grateful in the midst of blessing, and to trust our faithful God and Father for the future, assured that no creature shall separate us from his love, since all creatures are so completely in his hand that without his will they cannot even move." (p. 34)

[9] Smith WJ. *Forced Exit—The Slippery Slope.* New York: Times Books, 1997; Quill TE. *Death and Dignity.* New York: WW Norton, 1993.

[10] Ephesians 6:12

[11] Pegels E. *The Origin of Satan.* New York: Random House, 1995.

[12] The first miracle was performed by Christ in response to the concerned plea of his mother on behalf of the guests at a wedding in Cana who were about to run out of wine, a physical need during a

time of celebration [John 2:1–11]. There was great merriment, and they had no more wine! We are not to be mistaken here: this was not wine for a religious rite. This was wine for drinking, for joy, for laughter, for physical well-being.

13. Peck, MS. *People of the Lie*. New York: Simon & Schuster: 1983.
14. The Bible refers to this obstinacy in caricature as God hardens the heart of Pharaoh [Exodus 7]; but we are reminded that "God has mercy on whom he wants to have mercy, and he hardens whom he wants to harden" [Romans 9:18]. Our hard-heartedness (Greek σκληροκαρδιαν "sclerocardian" thus may not be entirely of our own volition, but when it is, it separates us from the love and promises of God.)
15. Berwick, DM, Hackbarth AD. Eliminating waste in US health care. *JAMA* 2012;307:1513–1516.
16. Brawley OW with Goldberg P. *How We Do Harm*. New York: St. Martin's, 2011.
17. Khatcheressian JL, Wolff AC, Smith TJ, et al. American Society of Clinical Oncology 2005 Update of recommended breast cancer surveillance guidelines. *J Clin Oncol* 2006;24:5091–5097.

5

Defeating Death for a Time

Domine Jesu Christe, Rex gloriae, libera animas omnium fidelium defunctorum de poenis inferni et de profundu lacu: libera eas de ore leonis, ne absorbeat eas tartaras, ne cadant in obscurum.[1]
—Mozart's *Requiem*, IV Offertorium

During my two years in the NHSC, I had the remarkable experience of participating in the successful resuscitation of a man who suffered a sudden cardiac arrest at a high school football game. This dramatic event reinforced my belief that death can sometimes be defeated. My clinical training had always focused upon overcoming death, but rarely did we learn how to usher patients and their families through the experience of dying with the same skill and confidence that we brought to our therapeutic endeavors. I would acquire those skills later both through personal tragedy and by caring for many dying patients in the years that lay ahead.

Nighttime entertainment is scarce in the hills of West Virginia. There are scattered "supper clubs" offering drinks and dancing, but the distances between homes and the clubs are vast, the bands are often bad, and the drive home after several hours of drinking is not an encouraging prospect to most patrons. Many individuals occupy themselves quietly during the long, dark West Virginia winter evenings. One of the reasons that arts and crafts and bluegrass music are so popular in the Appalachians is related to the social function they perform. There is no need for big-city entertainment if you are quilting or sewing, square dancing or picking a banjo with friends.

What about the kids? How do you keep them busy so they don't fall into more mischievous pursuits? The solution, for three months of the year in Nicholas County and many other civic-minded communities, was football. West Virginians are as enthusiastic about football as anyone in America. Towns all over the state have built elaborate stadiums for their high schools. They spare no expense to outfit their players, cheerleaders, and bands.

How does a rural school district in a poor state raise the grand sums that are required to fund a large athletic program? Higher school taxes were certainly not the solution, as they would have met opposition from those who could afford them and default from the many who would have been unable to pay. How, too, does the school board enlist the community to take ownership of the team and the band to ensure support throughout the year? The answer came through selling shares in the team, by selling multiple small pieces of the enterprise to those who would benefit from its use, the community itself. The solution also required that the path to shared ownership pay dividends to attract the shareholders in sufficient numbers.

The payment of dividends to its supporters was one of the most ingenious schemes ever devised for a local school district. The businessmen of Nicholas County—coal mine owners and equipment owners and operators—formed a sports association. Each year in the middle of winter, when the sun set at 4:45 p.m. in the local hollers and woodstoves warmed houses day and night, the sports association held its annual banquet. Every business in the Summersville community and throughout the county sold tickets for $50 each. There was nothing unique about that, although the price seemed high to me for a rural mining community. That, though, was only half the story. The enticement, the real hook that annually brought in tens of thousands of dollars to the Nicholas County athletic program, was that half the proceeds were shared with the banquet attendees by means of a lottery drawing that went on throughout the annual Saturday evening event.

Hundreds attended the festivities, and each diner bought at least one numbered entry ticket. Most who came bought more than one ticket, and some bought dozens. As soon as everyone sat down to dinner, the drawing of ticket numbers began, one at a time in a backward progression. It was an elimination drawing so that the numbers drawn were the losers, not winners. A huge tote board posted all the numbered tickets behind the head table. Next to each number was the owner's name, initials, or a code name. It seems that some attendees were too modest or too sensitive to have their names divulged. As the barker drew and announced each number, his assistants crossed the losing numbers off the tote board.

All through dinner we glanced repeatedly at the board to check our status between courses of the meal and its idle conversation. In keeping with the high spirits of the event, we feigned surprise when we recognized our last remaining number being called. Near the end of the meal, as fewer numbers remained on the board, everyone turned their attention to the barker, and all conversation ceased. At that point, where half the revenues had been retained by eliminating numbered tickets, the payoffs began. First, the payoffs were $50, the cost of the dinner. The $100 payoffs followed. There were dozens of these, and the winners smiled appreciatively as the barkers called their numbers and the tension mounted through the hall because the top payment was $5,000, and there were $1,000 and $2,500 payoffs on the way to the grand prize.

The feeling in the room for the last half hour of the drawing was like waiting for a baby to be born. Grown men literally paced as the numbers were called, and women wept, demonstrating either true ownership of this tradition by the community or true regret at suffering a financial loss at yet another sports banquet. Great adulation came from all as the organizers finally announced the winner, and community residents repeatedly talked about the evening and its festivities throughout the ensuing year until it was time to start selling tickets for the next event. This single event funded all the athletic programs in the high school and junior high school each year.

The ownership acquired by the community each year at the lottery banquet carried over every autumn through community-wide support and attendance at the high school's Friday night football games. The funds from the lottery built a huge lighted stadium in Summersville, and the scene on five Friday nights each fall rivaled those I later witnessed in Texas.[2]

As a newcomer to the community, it was impossible not to be captivated by the enthusiasm that all the residents expressed for the football team. The hospital administrator even told Sally and me about it during our recruitment interviews. Our real estate agent mentioned it. Even though Sally and I missed the chance to have a financial stake in our first football season because we missed the winter lottery, we eagerly anticipated the season opener. The entire spectacle brought back vivid memories of my playing high school football years earlier.

The Circles Narrow

I was not an accomplished athlete by any measure of my imagination. My athletic abilities were, on my best day, modest, but I had great admiration for the athletic heroes of my boyhood: Johnny Unitis, Bart Starr, Jim Brown, Ray Berry, and Lydell Mitchell. They were men to emulate, so at a strapping weight of 155 pounds, I was determined to play high school football.

It was hard work. Practices were long and hot, and physically demanding, with the very real possibility of getting hurt always present. I played in Pennsylvania, where the sons of coal miners and factory workers used the football field as a foundry in which to forge their manhood. We ran (yes, ran and seldom passed) old, forgotten formations with names like the "power I" and the "single wing T." The plays themselves had cast-iron names like "46 power" and "25 trap." We played on fields strewn with rocks and pieces of glass, with center crowns worn bare by cleats of players and the feet of countless band members. Lights were uncommon, lighted scoreboards rare, and the spectators sat on wooden bleachers surrounded by the spectacular colors that emblazoned autumn in southwestern Pennsylvania. We wore plain uniforms without stripes or leggings.

We were taught just to worry about beating the other guy, that player from the other team across from us. We focused on winning by executing our assignments as perfectly as we were able, just as they were diagrammed in the playbook. We learned that if we did our jobs, if we pulled our weight as a member of the team, we would win. When we lost, the coaches told us it was because our opponents had done their jobs better than we had done ours. My coaches instilled the virtues of teamwork, pride, sacrifice, and perseverance. We believed in them, and we won as a team. It all sounds just a little bit corny now, but in three years, I played on two championship teams. I played with accomplished, all-district athletes and with a future US congressman.

Our games generated palpable excitement in the school and in the community. The games were community events, talked about in barbershops, at the American Legion and the Elks Club, in stores and businesses. Our school was old-fashioned enough to have pep rallies, and our classmates were eager to attend, even as the society around us struggled with its ambivalence toward the war in Vietnam and discarded traditional virtues. We wore letter sweaters and the school colors, we had short hair, and we called the coach "Sir." We belonged to the town who owned us proudly. People came to our games day and night, home and away, in rain and snow. The local newspaper reported on us, and games were broadcast on the local AM radio station. The games represented all the performance and production that the young people and coaches of a small Appalachian town could muster. There were marching bands, majorettes, and cheerleaders. We had a homecoming with floats and a parade. It was thoroughly American.

I did not always play on the first team, although I was the starting end in some games. When I did not start, I had time to reflect on what was going on around us. I learned how to get glimpses of my family and friends in the stands without actually turning and looking at them (which would have been unacceptable to my game-hardened teammates and coaches). I could hear the cheerleaders and would peek over my shoulder at the majorettes to find the girl I was dating. I delighted at both the sounds of the band and the roar of the crowd. We lived for those games each week.

Robert Braugher, our coach, who was like many others of the era, often said in a tired athletic cliché that the game of football was like life, that what you did on the football field would carry on into whatever you did for the rest of your life. That sentiment came under attack in the 1960s along with a number of other cherished maxims, but I observed one similarity with some of the most profound experiences I had later as a physician. When I left the sidelines and entered the game, my world suddenly contracted upon itself. The multiple sensory inputs that I got from the crowd, the band, the cheerleaders, and the majorettes all disappeared on the field as if they had never existed. My world became a box one hundred yards long and fifty-two yards wide. The most important person in my world suddenly became the snorting behemoth lined up across from me, followed in importance by the tackle at my side and the barking of the quarterback, who started everything happening. At the snap of the ball, all disappeared except the man who was my assignment or the pass route that I tried to run as precisely as it was diagrammed. Everything else evaporated from consciousness. There was no crowd noise, no band, not even players and coaches on the sidelines. My world contracted suddenly and violently with each play.

That sphere could get even smaller.

Football is a rough game, even at the high school level, and young, strong bodies move very fast. Because of cleats and turf and the simple physics of the anatomy of human limbs, the violent collisions of a football game place stresses on joints they were never designed to withstand. Knees are particularly vulnerable, and I was not immune. During the last two weeks of August we practiced twice a day, starting at 8:00 a.m., stopping at 11:00 a.m., and starting again at 2:00 p.m. We hit two-man and seven-man blocking sleds in the summer heat, and we pushed heavy canvas blocking bags up and down the dusty, sometimes muddy, practice field. We listened to "chalk talks" about strategy, we were praised and criticized, and we became a team.

One Thursday morning during the intense two-a-day preseason workouts of late August, I was engaged in the routine drills of our practice session. We had practiced rushing the punter, and I had some success getting to the ball from my end position. We had also done sideline tackling drills, learning to get our heads in front of a runner sprinting down the sideline so as not to miss the tackle. We practiced this in small groups with much input from the coaches, and all had gone well.

We then came together as a team to practice tackling drills designed to teach us how to pursue a runner laterally along the line of scrimmage, squaring off at the last instant to make the tackle. Most of us played both offense and defense during the games, so everyone practiced on both sides of the ball. We lined up one-on-one, facing each other about five yards apart. One player carried a football, and the other was the pursuer. At the sound of the coach's whistle, the ball carrier broke to his left, turning up field around a blocking bag laid on the ground about five to seven yards from the starting point. The tackler's job was to get to the corner first and pop the ball carrier as he rounded the corner.

On my first attempt as the tackler, I just plain missed the runner. I set up to make the tackle too far inside the corner, I didn't square off and "break down," as they say in football lingo, and the runner stepped around me to the outside. That was the whole point of the drill: to keep the halfback from getting to the outside of the field.

I was angry with myself when I missed, and I told the coach I wanted to repeat my turn immediately. He agreed, and the running back and I lined up in our ready positions. I broke to my right at the first shrill sound of the whistle's blast and got to the bag ahead of the halfback, but only just ahead. As I planted my right foot to stop my lateral progress and turned to meet the halfback squarely, he turned up field, lowered his shoulders, and blasted me at full speed before I could lift my right foot and begin driving my weight into him. My turn to the left was accentuated by the force of his contact with me, but my one-inch cleats held my foot firmly in the sod. As he drove against me, my torso was forced violently to the left while the lower half of my right leg was angled to the outside at an ever-increasing angle. The force was more than my right knee could bear, and the collision tore both the medial and lateral cartilages and fractured the proximal tip of my right fibula.

All of this seemed to occur in slow motion—everything, that is, except for the pain, which came suddenly and monstrously, engulfing not only my knee, but my entire body. In an instant the pain was concentrated in my knee, but then it seemed to be everywhere simultaneously. I clutched my crippled joint, screaming and writhing in pain.

Suddenly, there was no world outside my right knee. There was no pride, no sacrifice, no valor—just pain. The pain was consuming and incapacitating, all-encompassing and total. As coaches rushed to attend me, I could barely feel their presence.

If they spoke, I could not hear. There was only the pain. My only thoughts were of my knee: Would it walk again? Would I heal? Could I play football again? Was I still on the team?

Gradually, the circle of my awareness widened as the pain ceased intensifying and merely remained constant. I began to see the coaches, to respond to their questions. They asked if I could stand, a curious question in retrospect. Why did they want me to stand? To my amazement I could stand, and within minutes I could walk. As the minutes passed, the circle of my consciousness continued to widen, and I could see teammates and the few spectators who were there to watch us practice.

"He's tough," said one of the fathers watching from the edge of the practice field.

I surely did not feel tough, but in a few weeks I was playing again, a fact that seems both miraculous and stupid years later. Eight months later in the spring of my junior year, the knee was surgically repaired. Playing on that wounded knee in the autumn it was damaged gave me the opportunity to injure it again and to witness the collapse of my sensory world around me into only the pain in my troublesome joint.

I have since come to know that the emotional response of the sick and dying to their psychic and physical pain is like the concentric collapse I witnessed on the football field when I felt extreme physical pain. The world of dying patients collapses around them, and their focus is limited to their pain and its relief.

The Circle Widens

The third home game of our first football season in Summersville was a tough defensive struggle. By the start of the fourth quarter, neither team had scored a touchdown. It was a beautiful, warm evening, and we all enjoyed the competitiveness of the game. I was sitting in the stands doing my best learning to root for the Grizzlies, having been in town only three months. Our gifted surgeon, Dr. Joo, was performing duties as team physician on the sideline, a task I later performed for the team during road games.

Late in the last period, Eric Moore, Summersville's talented halfback, eluded defenders and raced forty yards into the end zone to secure the win for a patient and appreciative home crowd. They had waited all night for something to cheer about, and the fans in the stands spared no emotion as students, parents, friends, and spectators screamed their exuberant approval.

As the cheering subsided after the successful point-after-touchdown, I noticed a great commotion among some of the fans to my left and several rows below our seats. I first thought that some kids were carousing or that someone had slipped off their seat during the excitement of the touchdown. A fight? A drunken fan? These seemed unlikely in our small, quiet town. As the gathered spectators slowly returned to their seats, I began to perceive a clearer image of the evolving drama, and the sight rivaled any made-for-TV medical show.

I recognized one of the hospital staff nurses with her arms locked in front of her, elbows fully extended in the rhythmic, controlled swaying that characterizes cardiopulmonary resuscitation. Another staff nurse knelt at the victim's head administering mouth-to-mouth resuscitation. People in the stands began to look at the frantic scene and realize someone was in serious trouble. I eased my way out of my row, stepping on feet as I hurried. Expectant eyes followed me, and someone asked, "What happened?" I responded politely that I couldn't tell from seventy-five feet away. What I found after I eventually made my way through the crowd to the concrete floor below the seats of Row 10 was controlled confusion. An elderly man was lying unconscious on his back as the nurses continued CPR.

"What happened?" I wondered aloud.

Susie Meadows, RN, slim and young and definitely in control, answered my question. "He fell onto us from the row behind during the touchdown. We thought he tripped, but then he turned blue. He wasn't breathing, and we couldn't find a pulse. So we started CPR."

The old guy got too excited, I told myself. Then someone yelled, "It's Coach Krieger's father!"

David Krieger was the backfield coach for the Grizzlies. He and his father, Dale, both lived in houses within sight of mine, and Dale never missed a home football game.

"Get Don Joo!" someone else yelled.

Don was already on his way up the stadium steps from the sidelines, but there wasn't much more a physician could do at that point other than continue the CPR. At the end of the field, I saw a man running toward an ambulance parked in the event of an injury to a player. The driver standing alongside nodded to the man, jumped into the ambulance, and drove on the track between the field and the stands, lights flashing with the siren off. Now everyone's attention was riveted on the unified effort to save Dale Krieger's life.

The game stopped. The stadium announcer asked that the spectators make way for the ambulance crew, and Don Joo and I watched the nurses skillfully do their jobs.

"I'll ride with you to the hospital," I told Don. "Someone should call the emergency room and let them know we're on the way." This was in the days before cellular phones; the ambulance drivers called on their radio.

The hospital was two miles from the field, and I was hoping that we would have a short, uneventful ride. Spectators in the stands made way for the ambulance crew to bring the litter up the stadium steps. I had never done CPR on steps before, but ambulance crews had told me spectacular tales about extricating victims from unimaginably small spaces, inclines, and holes, all while performing CPR. Some of the patients even lived!

So we kept it going, maintaining that rhythm all the way down those ten rows of steps to the ambulance. Don and I clambered inside ahead of the stretcher as the paramedics wheeled it in and locked the wheels. We tried desperately to continue the mechanics of the CPR through all the moving about. I held the mask of the Ambu bag tightly against Dale's face, squeezing the bag quickly after every five of Don's chest compressions.

The drivers turned the siren on and worked their way through the turf parking lot, gathering speed as they cleared the rows of parked cars. Autumn rains had soaked the parking lot before games earlier in the season. Now in the cool, dry days of early October, the solid ridges of the dried tire ruts caused us to bounce wildly inside the ambulance. We struck one rut so hard that Don and I were catapulted off our seats, Don's head hitting the ceiling as he flew. Somehow, we continued the CPR.

We accelerated rapidly when the ambulance finally reached the highway. Don and I worked in rhythmic succession, and the paramedics glanced at us occasionally with worried eyes through the sliding window that separated the front seat from the stretcher bay.

They know about Bob Fredrickson, I told myself fearfully. *They know the young hotshot doctor from the big-city hospital couldn't save one of the community's finest businessmen. Now he's going to lose the coach's father!*

I was haunted by the thought of another failure within three months of my arrival in Summersville. I believed that it was my skills, my decisions, that would determine if Dale Krieger lived or died. A small part of that belief was true. If you do things wrong as a doctor, people can and do die. As the years passed after that event, however, I learned a much harder lesson. You can do everything right, just as the books say to do, just as any expert would do on his best day, and the patient can still die.

That realization brought me to wrestle with questions that physicians and patients face only at the fringes of technology and medical knowledge. Where do we turn when the technology fails? If we stake all our hopes and trust on technological solutions, our confidence will fail when the technology cannot deliver a cure. A patient or physician with a spiritual history, with a faith, can turn to God, but what recourse is there for the patient who neither knows God nor understands the very real and finite limits of technology to deliver a solution? Such a patient and his family will be profoundly disappointed at the failure of the system, and these failures are known and documented since antiquity in the annals of medical science and religious literature.[3]

In many cases this disappointment leads both to frustration and litigation. As I look back on this situation years later, my foolish pride is evident. What did it really matter if I had done everything I was trained to do and this man died? Would my reputation suffer that seriously? Pride told me that people might consider me incompetent, yet I did not question my own competence. I eventually learned by carefully observing the expectant understanding shown by grieving families that they recognized I had done all I could, yet my diligent, competent efforts could not save their loved one.

We arrived at the hospital in less than five minutes, and the emergency room staff was awaiting our arrival. As Don and I continued CPR, we wheeled Dale into the treatment room, where the nurses quickly attached the electrocardiogram leads. The electronic tracing began to appear on the cardiac monitor, and we observed that Dale's heart was in ventricular fibrillation, an uncoordinated, quivering contraction of the heart muscle that results in ineffective pumping of blood and very low blood pressure. I asked the nurse in charge to give sodium bicarbonate and lidocaine through the intravenous line the paramedics had started at the stadium. There was no change in the cardiac rhythm after we gave the drugs. The charge nurse reported his blood pressure was 80 mm Hg systolic with each chest compression.

I picked up the defibrillator paddles from the table next to the stretcher and dialed in the highest energy setting: 400 watt-seconds. I placed the paddles on Dale's chest, asked everyone to clear the table, and hit the fire button. *Whompf!* Dale's chest heaved upward violently with the sudden transfer of energy. The cardiac monitor went blank as the electronic circuitry protected it from the defibrillating energy. Slowly, the tracing reappeared—regular sinus rhythm! This was a landmark moment in my young clinical career. I had performed successful cardiopulmonary resuscitation before, but never for a man whom I observed to have a cardiac arrest outside the hospital.

My elation was short-lived, however. The ventricular fibrillation returned after several minutes. We administered another bolus injection of lidocaine and reapplied the cardioversion paddles. *Whompf!* The energy jolted Dale's chest again, and again the normal cardiac rhythm returned. I asked the nurse to start a continuous infusion of lidocaine.

The three nurses who had resuscitated Mr. Krieger at the stadium soon arrived. Coach Krieger and his family followed quickly; the coach looked ashen.

"Dad has a history of heart trouble," he told me. "Three years ago, he was in the hospital in Charleston with abnormal heart rhythms. They had to shock him over and over. How's he doin', Doc?"

"We got his heart beating regularly again," I answered, "but I don't know how much damage was done. I don't know whether he's had a heart attack or whether there was any brain damage during the resuscitation. We will have to do some more blood tests and monitor his electrocardiograms."

"Should we take him to Charleston?" asked the coach.

It was a perfectly reasonable question, and I would have asked it myself had the patient been my father. I would hear it repeatedly during the years I was in Summersville. In the first few months, it rankled me because I felt people were questioning my abilities. The more I tried to put myself in the position of the patients, though, the more I agreed that they should question my abilities until I proved to them that I possessed sufficient skills to secure their confidence. As the months passed, I began to understand that there was an even greater reason to win the trust of the residents of this rural community. They needed to believe in their hospital; they needed to believe in its facilities and in its physicians, its nurses, and its support staff. They also needed to understand what it took me a very long time to learn: that large, technically sophisticated buildings and facilities alone do not deliver excellent health care. Excellent health care comes from well-trained individuals rendering sound, compassionate treatment in a setting where the welfare of the patient is the most important outcome.

Families and patients themselves often get confused about this. They equate elaborate technology with desirable, optimal health care, but technology is neither warm nor personal, and its use never assures a satisfactory outcome. There are illnesses, certainly, where technological solutions are desirable, such as cancer chemotherapy and stem cell transplantation, kidney dialysis, cardiac bypass surgery, intensive care nurseries, and the like. We have lost our way, however, in the morass of the technological jungle, and we have deluded ourselves into thinking that technology is the answer to all of our medical problems. In my experience, it is useful and even lifesaving for some patients. For most patients, though, very simple solutions will bring satisfactory outcomes.

"He's too sick to survive the ride to Charleston," I answered the coach. "If his heart stops on the way, he might not make it." As I said these words, terrifying visions of Bob Fredrickson jumped in my head. I wondered if Dale's family had similar recollections.

The coach reluctantly agreed. "Look," he said. "There's something you need to know. When Dad was in the hospital the last time, he was allergic to one of the medicines they gave him. It just made him crazy, and he got real agitated. I thought you better know that."

I thanked the coach as I puzzled over which medication he was describing. I checked with the nurses, who said that Mr. Krieger was already becoming so combative that they had to restrain him.

We had a two-bed intensive care unit in the hospital with monitored beds and arrhythmia alarms immediately adjacent to the nurses' station. We wheeled Mr. Krieger to the bed closest to the door. It took four of us to move him from the stretcher to the bed because he was a huge man. Within minutes of restraining him in the bed, Dale became extremely combative. He tore his leg restraint. He pulled at his nasal oxygen prongs. Debbie, one of the staff nurses, asked me if I thought he was allergic to the lidocaine, but I had never seen a lidocaine allergy that made a patient become combative.

"Can't be," I said aloud as I wondered silently if it could be. As the minutes passed, Dale remained physically agitated. I paced the floor. I sent the coach and his family home so they wouldn't see how anxious I was. After all, this was the same bed where Bob Fredrickson had died less than three months before. I didn't want to repeat that scenario. I looked in the *Physician's Desk Reference* to see if lidocaine caused restlessness and confusion. It said that it could. Why hadn't I seen this reaction in a patient before, during many months of training in coronary-care units? I was reluctant to stop the drug because his cardiac rhythm remained normal while he was stable, with only an occasional extra beat.

What if I stop it and he fibrillates again? I could lose him! I told myself. This was agonizing to me, and I realized how much agony his family must be in with this young, anxious doctor looking after their loved one. I was glad I was the doctor and not the family.

After much discussion with the nurses, we stopped the lidocaine and began procainamide, a reasonable alternative drug. Although Dale still did not wake up immediately, his restless thrashing ceased. By now, it was midnight. I dictated an admission note on the hospital transcription system and wrote admission orders. I admonished the nurses to call me if anything changed. I then realized that I did not have my car at the hospital because I had arrived by ambulance. I called Sally, and she arrived in less than ten minutes. I recapped the details of the previous two hours to her, and she easily sensed my concern. She assured me I had done all I could, and now we had to wait and let God do the rest. That was true, I agreed, but not easy to do.

The nurses called several times during the night with vital signs and the results of Dale Kreiger's cardiac rhythm tracings. He seemed stable and unchanged.

I got to the hospital by 8:30 a.m. Saturday morning. Dale was resting comfortably, but he was not awake. His son, the coach, arrived early, too, still worried. I repeated Dale's physical examination and found nothing changed. I compared his morning electrocardiogram with the one from the previous night and saw no signs of an acute myocardial infarction. His blood pressure was normal, even a little high, and his kidneys were working without evidence of any damage caused by low blood pressure during the resuscitation.

I wished there was something more I could do, but what was there? Even if we had been in a tertiary teaching institution, there would be little more to do, at least little more that would affect the outcome. After explaining the situation to the coach, I went home reluctantly, frustrated that I could do no more for this man. I knew that if I sat down and wallowed in my frustrations, I would have a perfectly miserable day. I reasoned with myself that some directed physical activity might get my troubled mind off the limits of medical technology.

Our house had unpainted cedar siding that was badly in need of some anti-weather treatment. My neighbor, Amos Preece, had sold me the house and advised me that it needed raw linseed oil to protect the cedar. I borrowed Amos's extension ladder, strapped my radio pager onto my belt, and started slapping the oil on the house with a coarse, wide brush. After a half hour, the beeper went off with its short, shrill beeps. *He has just died,* I told myself cynically.

Then, nurse Linda Queener's voice broke through the overcast of that gray October day and virtually shouted at me over the voice pager. "Dr. Vogel! I just wanted to let you know that Mr. Krieger is alert and awake, and he wants to talk to you!"

In my excitement, I narrowly avoided falling off the ladder. I was certain I had just participated in a miracle.

After I arrived at the hospital, Dale lucidly recounted his recollections of the events during the fourth quarter of the football game. When he was awake and cogent, he said that he had only one question for me (he actually had many). I told him that I would answer whatever questions he might have. "Doc," Dale asked, "Did that boy score the touchdown?" I assured Dale that he had.

He had made me smile, and he eased some of my self-absorbed anxiety. I joked that like him, most of the people at the game didn't know whether Eric had scored, thanks to all the commotion Dale had caused.

Amazingly, on the fifth hospital day, we sent him home quite well and robust once again.

Six months later in a ceremony in the hospital's visitors' lounge, the American Heart Association presented its Phoenix Award to Linda Queener, Marcia Farthing, and Susie Meadows for their lifesaving efforts in the successful resuscitation of Dale Krieger. We had bolstered the community's trust in the hospital by showing dramatically that what works best in health care are trained, conscientious people doing their jobs without a great deal of fanfare. I educated myself with that revelation.

The result of Dale Krieger's recovery and discharge from the Summersville Memorial Hospital was a sense of ownership by the community of their health care facility, the same sort of ownership they claimed for their high school football team. To validate that ownership meant to verbalize it publicly. Coach David Krieger and I did that in a letter to the Nicholas *Chronicle* shortly after the event. Coach John "Butch" Powell acknowledged the alert and speedy reaction of the staff nurses in his weekly *Chronicle* sports column. These written affirmations, accompanied by countless verbal retellings of the events of that Friday night by those individuals who were in attendance, led to a wider acceptance of the hospital as a trustworthy source of health care.

In a small way, this renewed public confidence began to repair years of pessimism and skepticism in the community about their hospital. This skepticism, often prevalent in America, is driven by the belief that "good health care" is highly technical, that it is delivered by subspecialists in tertiary referral hospitals, that it is expensive, and that it is our "right" to receive it. It is true that for some patients and their families, receiving highly specialized, technical care is a talisman that improves their self-worth and offers proof to the community that "we did all we could." The search for the magical—and frequently elusive—cure, however, often sends families in search of care far from home, depleting their emotional reserves and rarely resulting in a superior outcome for the patient.

The consequences of our search for highly technical medicine are the impediment of delivery of adequate, competent care at community hospitals and a burgeoning fiscal crisis in our national health care system. Ownership of health care by communities means that they will recognize the value of primary health care for the majority of their medical problems. They will obtain that care for themselves by supporting the health care providers in their community, and they will live with the assurance that, if the need arises, they will be able to obtain more sophisticated care at a referral hospital outside their community. This strategy requires education of the public and meticulous continuing medical education for the professional medical and nursing communities. It is a reasonable step toward reducing the inordinate costs associated with our often delivering primary care at tertiary institutions.

---

1   "Lord Jesus Christ, King of glory, deliver the souls of all the faithful departed from the pains of hell, and from the deep pit. Deliver them from the lion's mouth lest hell swallow them, lest they fall into darkness" Mozart's Requiem, IV Offertorium (No. 8, Domine Jesu) New York: CBS Records, 1986
2   Bissinger, Harry Gerard. *Friday night lights: a town, a team, and a dream*. Reading, MA: Addison-Wesley Reading, 1990.
3   "She had suffered a great deal under the care of many doctors and had spent all she had, yet instead of getting better she grew worse." (Mark 5:26).

6

Lifeguard: Death in the Family

> Civilian air ambulance flights responding to medical emergencies (first call to an accident scene, carrying patients, organ donors, organs, or other urgently needed lifesaving medical material) will be expedited by Air Traffic Control when necessary. When expeditious handling is necessary, add the word "LIFEGUARD" in the remarks section of the flight plan.[1]
> — Airman's Information Manual, "Aircraft Call Signs"

Nothing is so distressing to any of us—but particularly to a physician—as illness in a family member. No physician wants to see a loved one suffer, yet family members often corner their physician-relative, present him with less than all the necessary clinical details (because they are not medically trained), and then seek clarification, additional facts, a diagnosis, a treatment recommendation, a prognosis, or possible alternatives to the recommendations they have received from their own doctors. This can be disconcerting to the doctor who wishes to assist the ill family member and also wants to earn the respect of the family by showing that he is being wise, knowledgeable, and compassionate. With incomplete information, though, rendered by a well-meaning relative who is often only partly informed himself, the situation creates a challenge for the physician, especially when the sick relative is a parent.

Both my parents were unique and special individuals, and the relationship I had with my mother was distinctive in many ways. She was with me in my early years when my father was in seminary and the seminary, in holding to ancient but sometimes inexplicable tradition, required that its married students live apart from their families. My father was, therefore, absent from my early years, and the bond that grew between my mother and me formed earlier than the one that came much later with my father.

She was a shy and humble woman, but always quietly proud of her children, and her shyness amused me at times. On the day I was awarded the Boy Scout God and Country medal, she stood with me in front of our church and was asked to pin the medal on my Scout shirt. Her hands shook so badly in her anxious self-consciousness that she could not close the clasp, and as I walked to my seat, I was afraid the medal would fall off my shirt and embarrass both of us. Fortunately, that did not happen, but the event embodies my memory of her shyness.

Through several childhood illnesses, she was my nurse as well as my mother. My interest in medicine and her work in nursing strengthened the bond between us as I grew older. Certainly I taxed her patience, though, with my many illnesses and injuries. By the time I left home for college at age eighteen, I had ruptured my spleen, torn my knee cartilage, suffered an ocular hemorrhage (medically, an anterior chamber hyphema), and endured a number of infectious illnesses related to my asplenia. These afflictions would have been a challenge for any mother, and mine was exasperated at times. When I finally reached adulthood in good health, she told me of a friend of hers who had lovingly reassured her that I would grow up to be a fine young man. That may have explained why she beamed at my college graduation, knowing that I was finally on my way to medical school, and, she hoped, finished with my childhood traumas.

My most cherished aspect of our relationship was what developed when I embarked on my medical career. As soon as she knew of my interest in medicine, she regaled me with stories from the hospital, of the daily drama that unfolded in those rooms and hallways. She kept her nursing textbooks in our hall closet, and I delighted myself for hours, turning the pages slowly as I pored over the photographs of the patients with exotic illnesses and the diagrams of complex surgical procedures. She seldom discussed the texts with me, but she didn't discourage my looking, either. When I graduated from college, Mother was quite delighted that I had chosen her field as my profession.

When I was in medical school, I made a habit of calling her every Friday evening to review the events of the week. She delighted in hearing my stories, and she shared with me the ongoing activities in her hospital. As we had these conversations, I could not imagine, nor could she, how our medical lives would intertwine so intimately or so fatefully in the years ahead. Neither could I envision the enormous effect that her coming illness would have on my perceptions of myself as a physician or on my understanding of the meaning of suffering and death.

I grew up in south-central Pennsylvania in the rich farmland that the German immigrant farmers transformed in the eighteenth and nineteenth centuries into some of the most productive farms in the world. The showcase was in Lancaster County, where the Amish maintained meticulously manicured properties without the benefit of powered machinery. For the residents of these rural farm communities, local medical practitioners provided health care in the 1950s and 1960s before the emergence of the large, technology-based modern hospitals that would follow them. When serious illness struck, families in eastern Pennsylvania traveled to nearby Philadelphia or Baltimore to find sophisticated care. When I was a boy, I marveled at the stories recounted by those who journeyed to Johns Hopkins or Hahnemann or the University of Pennsylvania and returned home mended and whole. A first-grade classmate of mine had gone to the Wilmer Eye Institute at Johns Hopkins after an errant arrow had amazingly found its way through the smallest of openings in a wooden shack and destroyed his right eye as he peered innocently at his playmates through a peephole. Even though he lost his eye, his family spoke fondly, almost reverently, of Johns Hopkins. My mother and father acknowledged that this hospital was a special place, and my curiosity grew as I repeatedly heard tales throughout my youth of this marvelous institution of learning in the "land of pleasant living," as announcer Chuck Thompson would say as I listened to Baltimore Orioles baseball games on the radio.

Perhaps because of my fantasies about the venerable institution to the south of my boyhood home, or perhaps simply by ironic coincidence, I received most of my education in the Johns Hopkins institutions, first as an undergraduate, then as a resident in medicine in one of its affiliate hospitals (now named the Bayview Medical Center), and finally as a fellow at both the hospital and in the School of Hygiene and Public Health. It turned out to be as wonderful as I had imagined it to be: large and grand and filled with some of the brightest and most gifted individuals I have ever met.

It was within this romantic and intellectual idealism that I entered and interacted with Johns Hopkins as a means to an end, my pathway to an academic medical career, and a great and significant part of my medical education. It was the embodiment of everything to me that was medicine: academic, compassionate, highly regarded, and regularly and repeatedly offering the dual products of educated health professionals and unequaled medical care for its patients. I experienced only excellence in the Hopkins institutions. All whom I encountered had the single-minded purpose of learning and giving the best possible medical care to their patients. Mother would not or could not utter the words that described her pride when I matriculated at Hopkins, but she was unquestionably and quietly proud. Curiously, from that pride I derived a sense of obligation to her that would follow me throughout our mutual and tragic journey that neither of us could foresee.

We were only twenty-five miles apart while I was in medical school at Temple University in Philadelphia. She was working as a medical/surgical head nurse at our community hospital in Norristown, Pennsylvania, when I spent a brief two-day surgical rotation at her hospital as a freshman medical student. As the years passed, our understanding and appreciation of each other grew continuously. She became my sounding board during my internship and residency. When I was tired and discouraged, she counseled me. She frequently reminded me that she was a nurse and I was a physician, and that there were differences between us that could not be bridged even by a mother and her son. Now, years later, I can see that her sentiments clandestinely embodied but did not openly acknowledge the medical chauvinism and paternalism that permeated her training. I wish she could have lived to see the changes that came in medicine that began to combat the inequity between nurses and physicians and between men and women. Her counsel and advice were always there for me, and she was fascinated and intrigued as she accompanied me with Dad on a tour of the Baltimore City Hospital during my internship.

Mom trained in the 1940s, before medicine experienced its modern technological explosion. She amazed me with stories from her early career about melting medications on spoons over alcohol lamps, and sterilizing hypodermic needles for reuse. She knew what I was becoming before I knew, and she quietly and gently reflected that knowledge and confidence as I slowly acquired competence and experience through my training. Our family, being stoic German Calvinists, did not speak often in explicit terms about our emotions or our feelings for one another, so Mother and I communicated our love for each other silently rather than explicitly between the lines of our conversations about medicine.

As I noted above, physicians are sometimes called on to counsel family members in medical matters and to make recommendations about diseases or illnesses in which they may not be expert. Often a doctor in the family can experience mild frustration if a relative confronts him with unrealistic expectations and much anxiety. This phenomenon is becoming less common, perhaps, in this age when patients increasingly employ a passel of specialists for their variety of illnesses, and family members now recognize that not all physicians are the same: a pediatrician is not an adult gastroenterologist. They can also buoy their knowledge on the Internet, for better or worse.

After I completed my medical oncology training at Johns Hopkins, I accepted a faculty position at the University of Texas M. D. Anderson Cancer Center in Houston. The distance between Houston and Pennsylvania complicated my opportunities to spend time with my mother except for one delightful fact of academic life. Academic medicine requires a great deal of travel, often to the East Coast. During October, shortly after our move to Houston, I was attending a meeting of one of the country's large breast cancer research groups (the National Surgical Adjuvant Breast and Bowel Project or NSABP) in Washington, DC. I was staying in the Embassy Row Hotel on Massachusetts Avenue, enjoying the prospect of new clinical research that would explore the possibility of preventing breast cancer along with the attractions of the nation's capital in autumn.[2]

During a breakfast meeting, I was interrupted by a front desk attendant who asked me to call my office in Houston urgently. My staff there told me that my father was desperately trying to contact me, and I called him at home immediately, fearing that something had happened to Mother. He advised me instead in his calm, pastoral voice that my grandmother had become gravely ill. He also told me somberly that my mother was fine, although distressed. After her breast cancer diagnosis years before, Grandma had developed colon cancer, a disease that may occur with greater frequency in some women with a prior diagnosis of breast cancer. Grandma was now quite ill, but Dad was not sure about the clinical details. I said I would fly from Washington to Bethlehem as soon as possible to help in any way I could. I wasn't sure whether he wanted me to come to interrogate the medical staff so that I could brief the family on her diagnosis and prognosis, or to see my grandmother in her final hours. Whatever the reasons, I thought I should get to the hospital in Pennsylvania as quickly as possible.

The USAir De Havilland Dash 8 commuter got me from Washington National airport to Allentown-Bethlehem-Easton airport in northeastern Pennsylvania in less than an hour. The route was a familiar one I had flown myself many times from Baltimore to Lancaster and on to ABE airport. The scenery elicited memories of a harrowing flight from Baltimore to ABE on my birthday several years earlier.

Sally and I planned to fly in our rented Beech Sundowner to celebrate my birthday with my parents and grandmothers. The wind was blustery out of the northwest, and the sky was crystal blue with only scattered cumulus clouds. The cold March Saturday morning was punctuated by a single snow shower that required us to deviate to the east just southwest of Reading. Allentown approach control vectored us to a visual approach to Runway 31, and the final approach took us over Bethlehem's South Mountain. The wind was brisk at twenty knots, gusting to thirty-five, but no turbulence was reported by approach control or by other aircraft in the area. Our flight had been smooth in spite of the fact that there was a Sigmet (an advisory for *sig*nificant *met*eorological conditions) for moderate to severe turbulence below 10,000 feet that I got from the Flight Service Station during my telephone weather briefing in Baltimore. Why we decided to go anyway is not at all clear in retrospect.

We were on a five-mile straight-in final approach, lined up for landing and descending out of 2,300 feet over the mountain with wings level when suddenly and without warning we plunged straight down at an enormous rate of speed. The severe downward acceleration lifted both Sally and me violently out of our seats. The microphone stored in the plane's center console flew upward and was momentarily suspended between us. My head smashed into the cabin roof, and only my shoulder harness prevented me from striking the roof hard enough to lose consciousness. Amazingly, the Sundowner continued in straight, descending flight and we landed without incident, although we were badly shaken. My chilly and windblown parents and both grandmothers were anxiously waiting for us in the frosty air as we taxied through the gusting wind. They were unaware of the danger that had stalked us over the mountain.

(An anticlimactic incident occurred on our return to Baltimore later in the afternoon when the alternator quit, eliminating our source of electrical current, and we made a no-radio approach into the Baltimore airspace, landing with light signals from the tower at Glenn L. Martin State Airport. The violent turbulence over the mountain had broken the armature rotor in the alternator, and the damage was not apparent until the battery failed.)

After I arrived in Bethlehem, I quickly learned that the situation was not good, nor was the scene in Grandma's hospital room a pleasant one. My family was overcome with tearful anxiety. My mother, two aunts, and an uncle were pacing about. My father had picked me up at the airport, and he and I left the room so that I could ask the nurse in charge whether it might be possible for me to look at Grandma's medical chart. It was there that I learned of her condition and the gravity of the situation. Grandma had experienced a local recurrence of her colon cancer that resulted in a bowel perforation. The perforation, in turn, led to bacterial sepsis, and she was near death, with low blood pressure and poor kidney function.

What was I to do? I struggled silently with myself for a moment and decided that I should speak the truth but try to infuse some hope into the situation. Her doctors were giving Grandma antibiotics, and her fever had subsided, but this was an eighty-four-year-old woman, and she had gained consciousness only briefly and intermittently since being admitted to the hospital.

St. Luke's Hospital in Bethlehem was special to our family. My sister and I were born there, my mother and her sisters went to nursing school there, and Sally and I had done fourth-year medical student externships there. Aunt Matilda, my mother's sister, had died there, and now the drama was being repeated again.

There was visible agony on the faces of all who were present in her room that morning. They turned to me for an interpretation of the situation rather than for answers, and I explained the circumstances as well as I could in lay language. The reversal of roles seemed peculiar to me because I was now serving as an authority for the extended family that had raised me, played with me, teased me, and guided me through childhood. They had sustained my nuclear family in my illnesses, and now I was, in a strange way, repaying a small portion of a substantial debt.

Was I the son, grandson, and nephew coming to grieve over his ailing and beloved grandmother, or was I the young academic physician swooping in on the latest commuter flight to save Grandma from avoidable death? The latter seemed possible, but I could not improve on the care being rendered. I explained the situation to my family. They seemed relieved to hear that my reading of Grandma's medical record yielded the same summary her physicians had presented to them earlier. I said that with the antibiotics, she had a chance of improvement, and that I had seen such recoveries in my clinical experience (limited as it was so early in my career). I boldly suggested that she could recover and return home in ten to fourteen days. I answered a few questions from my relatives, walked to the bedside, held Grandma's hand, and leaned over to her. I kissed her cheek and whispered, "I love you, Grandma," and she mumbled, "I love you too" in return.

I tried to be optimistic, as I always am with families at the bedside, but my own family could sense my concern through even my most crafty bedside aptitudes. I realized suddenly that I could not make my family believe what I did not believe myself. This simultaneously agitated and horrified me. My mother was particularly annoyed with me when I suggested that Grandma could recover. Now the nurse was educating the doctor, and I was frustrated with my inability to offer any additional solace to her at such a difficult time.

My mother followed me into the hall, where she confronted me.

"You don't really think she is going to go home, do you?"

"I have seen it happen, Mother," I reassured her, and I had.

"Even if she does recover from the sepsis," she protested, "it will be weeks before she can go home!"

I was confused. Was I being questioned by a senior nurse, which Mother certainly was, or by a distraught family member who had lost her beloved sister to cancer and who was about to lose her mother in the same way? It is not easy to reassure people in pain, especially if they see no end to their suffering, if they are fearful for themselves, and if the messenger is someone they perceive to be as vulnerable as themselves. I had been able to convince families before that all would be well and that a loved one would recover, but I couldn't bluff Mother. She knew medicine too well, knew when I had unexpressed doubts, and knew from her own experience that many elderly patients who are this ill do not recover.

I simply said, "We'll see," kissed my mother good-bye, and returned to the airport.

As I flew home to Houston, my rational, clinical self told me that I would soon return to celebrate Grandma's life at her memorial service. Our hope would not change the reality of her illness, and the healing we prayed for would come in a way we did not want. Grandma died a few days later, and I felt a bit foolish for having been too optimistic at her bedside. What I meant to show was hope that was deeper and more profound than just optimism. When I saw my mother again, she made me understand that she fully understood my concern for Grandma, but she also let me know that she was not about to be the fool who naively believed that all would be well just because the family's young doctor said so. This was a lesson for me that was both painful and humbling, belittling and necessary.

My father conducted the memorial service for his mother-in-law. As always, his liturgical gifts graced the morning. He had a special relationship with Grandma, and he always called her "Naoma" as he spoke to her in her kitchen or ours. His sermon that bright October morning was about the legacy of faith she had left to four generations, and about how we would all carry on the legacy because of her. He was a remarkable comfort to all of us.

I rarely saw Mother cry, but she wept openly at the cemetery as Grandma's casket was lowered into the vault. Mother changed with Grandma's death. She was never as happy again, nor was she ever very optimistic. Grandma had been her best friend in many ways, and they had lived only a few miles apart. They saw each other several times during a typical week. They shopped together, went to church together, and talked often. Mother said that after Grandma died, she once picked up the telephone and began to dial her number before suddenly realizing she was no longer there. We closed an entire chapter of our family history the morning Grandma was buried, not knowing or suspecting that more difficult times would follow.

Soon, tragedy struck again.

Mother's Breast Cancer

Years before Grandma's death, Mother had scared me during my freshman year at college. She called to tell me that she had a lump in her breast and that she needed to undergo a biopsy. Her aunt had had breast cancer years earlier, but she was doing fine, and Mother did not seem terribly afraid. I knew, though, that she did not always share emotions well. I also knew in 1970—even before going to medical school—that a breast biopsy was a harrowing experience for a woman, even more than it is now. Those were the days before Rose Kushner created the two-stage procedure, when a patient woke up not knowing whether she had benign fibrocystic disease and only a small scar on the breast or had had a mastectomy for breast cancer.

I knew then, even at age eighteen, that this was extremely distressing for Mother. I would learn years later how much anxiety is generated for a person who is medically knowledgeable when they undergo any procedure, because they know, unlike the unsuspecting layperson, of numerous possible outcomes of any diagnostic venture, and that at least some of those outcomes have dire implications and consequences. This is what Mother referred to when she said, "Ignorance is bliss," or "What you don't know can't hurt you." Mother used to entreat me with a number of her aphorisms, such as "Self-praise stinks." Earthy, unpolished, and true. It is true that denial (or ignorance) works for a time. There is temporary bliss in our not knowing the possible implications of certain pathological features of a cancer diagnosis.

Mother meant that patients who are medically unwise need not know all the terrible possibilities that medical professionals know explicitly. This is changing somewhat in the current litigious climate that requires exhaustive (and often unnecessarily frightening) informed consent procedures, but I would rather be a slightly less knowledgeable layman facing major surgery than a trained medical professional who reads the medical literature and grasps the probability of dying or of injury with quantifiable mathematical certainty.

Mother's call about her breast biopsy created for me my first personal awareness of the battle Christian physicians fight all of their professional lives in regard to their faith and the health of those they treat. After Mother called, I desperately wanted to pray for her. I cannot remember whether I wanted to pray that she be well or that God would give her the strength to face her ordeal. I probably hoped for both. My struggle was with my roommate, an acknowledged agnostic who openly expressed his annoyance at my church attendance and my daily devotions. He challenged me with great examples of his intellectual prowess by posing such philosophical challenges as "Vic, prove to me that you exist!" At age eighteen, I found that distressing; I now find it both trite and amusing that a visible, physical being requires abstract, philosophical validation.

With great reluctance and some embarrassment, I hit my knees in my college dormitory that autumn evening and asked God to spare my mother. I did it silently but openly, and I am sure that I selfishly included a request on my own behalf that God not take my mother from me. I was a bit ahead of myself in my anxiety, because we did not even know that she had breast cancer, and the prayer was imperfect in that it equated my anxieties about my mother's health with her health itself. I do acknowledge, though, that such a multi-tiered request is acceptable, for what young man would not pray that his mother be spared, if only to preserve his relationship with her and not simply to relieve her pain?

I do not know what effect my prayer had on my roommate, and I never intended it to be a conscious witness of my faith. It was meant only as a fervent supplication to God on behalf of my mother. If my roommate concluded that I loved my mother greatly, he was right. If he also concluded that I was somewhat primitive and unintellectual in my thoughts and beliefs, then he did me the service of introducing me to unbelief at an early age. My struggle with the unbelief of others has been ongoing in the dual aspects of my intellect and faith since that moment.

Mother's biopsy was benign, but I failed to convince my agnostic roommate that faith was a tenable option when confronting suffering. Years later, as I observed families praying fervently that their loved one be saved, I realized that when we pray for a loved one, we are usually praying for ourselves. Yes, we want God to spare our loved one, but what we really want is for God to spare us the agony of our own suffering in the loss of our loved one. It is extraordinarily difficult to make supplication for another when we cannot calm our own fears or ease our own pain.

For ten years all was well. Then, while I was in residency training, my grandmother and aunt, Mother's mother and sister, both received a diagnosis of breast cancer. We all knew that the diagnosis in these family members greatly increased Mother's chance of developing breast cancer at some time in her life. Tragically, as I completed my residency training, my aunt's breast cancer advanced rapidly, and she died during my first month in the US Public Health Service. My mother was very close to her sister and was devastated by her death. Mother became maudlin in her predictions that she would be the next in the family to get a diagnosis of colon cancer. I tried weakly to convince her otherwise, but it was impossible for the two of us to hide in that blissful ignorance that neither one of us could embrace. At times as I talked to her before her diagnosis, I could sense Mother's fatalism about her inevitably developing breast cancer, and her resignation angered me greatly. I never expressed my anger to her because medical training teaches physicians to swallow emotion, and I, myself, could not dissuade Mother of her pessimism. So we danced a waltz of silent anger, waiting for the inevitable.

---

[1] Airman's Information Manual, Paragraph 4-2-4, "Aircraft Call Signs." U. S. Department of Transportation Regulations, Aeronautical Information Manual, 1995. In 2012, the term *Lifeguard* was replaced by the term *MEDEVAC*. Because of the priority afforded air ambulance flights in the ATC system, extreme discretion is necessary when using the term *MEDEVAC*. It is intended only for those missions of an urgent medical nature and to be used only for that portion of the flight requiring expeditious handling.

[2] During the visit, I had breakfast with a consultant friend of mine, and while we were meeting, former senators Gary Hart and George McGovern took a table near us in the dining room. Although it was not an election year, Ellen and I strained to overhear the strategies that these two defeated politicians might be crafting during their conversation. Sadly, we could hear nothing.

7

Through a Glass Darkly

> When I was a child, I talked like a child, I thought like a child, I reasoned like a child. When I became a man, I put the ways of childhood behind me. For now we see only a reflection as in a mirror; then we shall see face to face. Now I know in part; then I shall know fully, even as I am fully known.
> —1 Corinthians 13:11–12

Fourteen years after her first breast biopsy, the second edition of my heartfelt supplication to quiet my fears and spare my mother's agony did not yield the desired result. It was while I was a medical oncology fellow at Johns Hopkins that the feared but perhaps expected outcome finally occurred. Mother called me at home one evening and said she had been to her surgeon, had a biopsy, and learned that she had breast cancer. Just like that: so matter-of-fact, so objective, and so unemotional. I think she was hiding her feelings purposefully to protect the family from our own pain, from our own unexpressed horrors that Mother would die painfully and suddenly as her sister had done. Mother's only evident bitterness was over the fact that her mammogram did not show her breast cancer a mere three or four months before her diagnosis. My ineffective explanations to her about false-negative examinations sounded hollow even to me.

Mother shared little with me about her expectations and fears as she went through with her surgery and post-operative chemotherapy. Her oncologists, after learning that I was a medical oncology fellow, were dutiful in their sending copies of her progress notes, and there was little I could add to their competent care. My father did an admirable job in helping her through her post-operative rehabilitation, and he showed no reluctance to change her chest dressings or to be a source of real comfort. For me, though, this troublesome ordeal showed me the limits of my abilities as an oncologist to do all that I wanted for someone I loved. After all, I was at Johns Hopkins, and I had believed since my boyhood that they (now we) could work miracles. It seemed now that none would be forthcoming, and I asked myself whether my faith was in the healing power of God or in the healing power of cyclophosphamide, methotrexate, and fluorouracil.

I made frequent trips home from Baltimore to Pennsylvania after Mother's diagnosis both to cheer her and to share her grandchildren with her. They were able to delight her more than I could. After Mother's diagnosis, there was an unspoken tension between us that persisted throughout her illness. It was as if she believed my colleagues and I had let her down, but she never expressed this thought, and I do not actually believe she even thought so. Nevertheless, as irrational as it was, I continued to think so. She would look at me and grin when she told me about her test results or about what her oncologist had said, as if she were expecting me to respond in some yet unexpressed way. I would find myself couching my responses in protective language that was more reserved and more measured than I would use with my own patients, and she would see right through it. *You can't bluff a nurse,* I told myself, and no matter how sophisticated and educated I might become, I certainly couldn't bluff my own mother.

Mother knew somehow that her prognosis was bad, although the odds were in her favor at the time of her diagnosis. She firmly expected, I believe, to repeat her sister's experience, and her pessimism clouded her outlook and her expectations. It is difficult for a physician to combat a patient's pessimistic outlook, and he can never really gain advantage over the patient psychologically. If I tell a patient she is fine and try to reassure her, she will say that, although that is true today, neither she nor I can possibly know what tomorrow will bring. If in the passing years she remains well, she can still have misgivings about her remote and still uncertain future. When the future ultimately yields disaster, the pessimistic fatalist will say, "I told you so!" and the physician is momentarily defeated. My only recourse in that situation is to remind the patient that I will not abandon her, and that I will struggle against every attack that the disease may bring upon her. I tell my patients that I will be their physician no matter what happens, but I could not be my mother's doctor; I could only promise to be her son.

Optimism was at times dreadfully difficult for me to maintain, and the situation only got worse when my grandmother got her diagnosis of colon cancer. Now there was yet more uncertainty, and there were more assaults to defend against. After her surgery, though, the questions began to come rapidly from both my mother and her, and once again, I found it difficult to be both honest and encouraging. The stage was set for disaster. This was the familial disease, and all of the women in the family were at risk, including my sister, who was only thirty-three years old at the time. Mother was surprisingly frank about the entire experience and accepted her plight with the sober resignation that our family knew all too well.

I was not so sanguine. For the first time in my professional life, I understood what distinguishes physicians from the laity: we are caretakers of special knowledge. We know facts that can help predict frightful and uncertain futures. This ability is not necessarily an advantage, because it burdens us with anticipatory grief that those with less knowledge can deny or at least delay. Those of us who carry that special knowledge are burdened with a view of future events that include multiple unattractive possibilities. This uncertainty about the timing and seriousness of future events generates anxiety for us because we know the ills that can afflict us. We recognize that our patients are uncertain about those ills and that their fantasies may be worse than the approaching reality of their illnesses. I even once, somewhat callously in a moment of pompous weakness that provided little comfort, told a patient's wife that she should be glad she did not know what I knew, because the knowledge was too painful. Perhaps that is so, and perhaps full disclosure is more compassionate, but predicting the future, even with special knowledge, is a precarious task. It is far better that I now tell my patients that I will walk with them through whatever challenges and obstacles we may encounter on our journey, including those we cannot foresee.

I am not sure that Mother knew fully the implications of her diagnosis, whether she knew what significance resided in the size of the tumor, the microscopic involvement of her axillary lymph nodes with metastatic cancer cells, or the absence of estrogen receptor protein in the primary tumor. She and I cautiously chose not to explore all the implications of her breast pathology, and we shared a peculiar emotional tango as we secretly explored each other's knowledge while avoiding questions that were too sensitive or too close to the reality of her diagnosis. She never asked me, for example, what percentage of patients with estrogen receptor-negative tumors and positive axillary nodes eventually relapse. She did ask me about her need for chemotherapy. When I offered my opinion that it was necessary, I must have confirmed her suspicions, but she never voiced them openly. I knew that she was aware of the somber implications of her diagnosis, but I did not want her to know what I knew as an oncologist, that the odds might not be in our favor.

I told myself that she had to know how deadly serious all of this was, and the implications of her diagnosis haunted me, as did the burden of my special knowledge. That knowledge allowed me to peer into the dark, anticipated future of someone I loved. I found myself wishing for miracles that I did not yet need while battling fears that would not abate in the presence of the facts. I offered Mother consultation at Johns Hopkins with my mentors, who were among the most knowledgeable breast cancer physicians in the country, but she and my father both declined. I actually knew that a consultation was unnecessary at this stage of her illness, and that she was getting adequate care from her community oncologists, but I felt I had to offer the possibility of a consultation lest I appear insensitive. Early in her illness, I falsely believed that my own ability to care for her suffering would occur only with medicine and not with the love that a son can give his mother. Eventually, that misperception would change.

After completing my medical oncology fellowship at Johns Hopkins Hospital and an Andrew W. Mellon Fellowship in clinical epidemiology at the Johns Hopkins School of Hygiene and Public Health (now the Bloomberg School), I moved our family to Houston. Sally and the children and I returned home for Christmas six months after our move to Texas, and Mother seemed well. She had lost her hair because of her chemotherapy, but she was still working as a nurse and her spirits were high, elevated even more by the presence of her grandchildren. For a time, optimism prevailed as we continued our shadow dance. "Ignorance is bliss" as Mother often said, even when we only pretend to be ignorant. I made frequent trips home to Pennsylvania after Mother's diagnosis both to cheer her and to share her grandchildren with her. They were able to brighten her more than I ever could alone.

After Mother's diagnosis, there was an unspoken tension between us, as if I had failed her, but she never expressed this openly. It is more likely that her pessimistic Calvinism consigned her to weak resignation to her fate. As irrational as it was, I continued to think we had, indeed, failed her, and I wished deeply that there was more we could do. She would look at me with her wry grin when she told me about her test results or what her oncologist had said, expecting me to respond in a predictable way. This is what I faced with Mother, and hopefulness was at times desperately difficult.

Recurrence

My parents made an annual visit to Houston each autumn. Just before their visit in 1989, Dad called me at home to explain that Mother's breast cancer had recurred on the skin of her chest. Fortunately, there was no evidence of involvement of any other organs in her blood work, scans, or X-rays. He explained that her oncologist had consulted with a radiation therapist who had begun treatment to her chest wall. Chemotherapy was planned to follow the completion of the radiation. I expressed my concerns for her and then inquired selfishly whether her treatment would be completed in time for their visit to Houston. Dad assured me that they would try to make the trip.

There are some words and phrases that, for a physician, evoke whole pictures of evolving scenarios that unfold as clinical dramas. *Recurrent breast cancer is* one of those phrases. After I had seen hundreds of breast cancer patients, it was obvious to me, as it is to any physician who deals with metastatic cancer, that the progression of the disease is often inexorable, that only palliation is possible, and that profound suffering is a distinct possibility. This clinical fast-forwarding that goes on in the mind of a clinician as he anticipates the future of his patient must be analogous to the phenomenon of having your life "flash before your eyes" or of "seeing things happen in slow motion" in the instant before a serious accident that is frequently recounted by recovering victims. My mother's whole life was now flashing before my eyes, and for the first time in my own life, I could see the end of hers in the distance. At that moment, I longed for some of that blissful ignorance that Mother and I had spoken of often, but it would not come. I had peered behind the magician's curtain too often, and I knew all his props. I knew that there was nothing in the bag of magic that could ultimately save Mother, and I desperately wished I knew differently. I wondered how Mother could possibly endure the burden of her own recurrent illness so soon after the death of her own mother. Who would provide her consolation? Who would be her friend and sounding board? Was hope still possible?

Yes, it was possible, but it had to be reframed with more realistic expectations. I could no longer anticipate a cure unless God in his providence chose to effect a miracle. Possible, but unlikely, my experience told me. My larger problem was how to interact with Mother after the experience with Grandma taught me that there would be no clinical charade here, no pretending with an empty hand of cards. Mother and I silently knew we were both in a death struggle, and that the enemy had more ammunition than we did.

It was difficult for me to see Mother face-to-face when she visited. It was not because we couldn't talk honestly. In fact, she asked me openly, "This is not good, is it?" I assured her reluctantly that it was not. It was difficult to see her in pain from the radiation burn on her chest. She was a fair-skinned redhead, and the radiation had caused painful erythema (skin redness) that was so uncomfortable, it was difficult for her to wear her clothes because the mere contact irritated her skin even more. I ached for her, but there was little to offer other than the narcotic analgesics her radiation oncologist had already prescribed. I was so grateful that my children continued to bring her some delight.

I began to sense that time was running out for our family. All the shared experiences would never be repeated; they were now just memories. Grandma was gone, and with her, the house where, for almost thirty years, we had had parties and picnics and laughed and sang and had been a family. Now, Mother was making preparations to leave, and I was haunted by a sense that my world was changing forever. *The seasons of a man's life,* I thought, *but I prefer spring to the bleak midwinter.*

Sally and I discussed our strategy for dealing with Mother's illness often during that autumn. It was easy for Sally as a physician to understand the gravity of the situation. We agreed that whenever I had business trips in the East, I would make an effort to get home to see Mom even if it meant extra days or expense.

By early the next spring, her bone scan showed widespread metastases, and she was struggling with increasing pain throughout her body. One morning, Dad called to say that he had taken Mother to the emergency room because her back pain had worsened, and the analgesia they had given her was not effective. I asked him to take her back to the emergency room. We got her pain under control. In June, I visited my parents and attended a congregational meeting with them at my father's church. After a two-year struggle, the congregation voted 135–11 in favor of constructing an addition to the church building. My parents were elated.

While all of this was going on, my academic career was on a meteoric track. My speaking and lecture schedule took me to New York, Washington, Paris, and Berlin during the year. I also had meetings and speaking engagements in Boston; Toronto; Atlanta; Olympia, Washington, and Winston-Salem, North Carolina. In mid-March, Dad and I managed to find time to hear the Bach Choir of Bethlehem perform the *St. John's Passion* in the Packer Memorial Chapel at Lehigh University. I met my sister, Louise, for a birthday dinner in Washington, DC. At national meetings with colleagues, my data were used to design future clinical trials. At a talk I gave at North Shore University Hospital on Long Island, I was introduced as "one of the young rising stars in oncology." I traveled to Boston for the sixth International Breast Cancer Conference, and I met with Drs. Judy Garber and Fred Li at the Dana Farber Cancer Institute to discuss my work.

In early October, I was invited to Dallas as one of the recipients of a Susan G. Komen Breast Cancer Fellowship. At the luncheon for the fellows and hundreds of prominent women from Dallas and the state of Texas, I met the first lady of Texas, Rita Clements; soon-to-be governor George W. Bush; former Dallas Cowboys coach Tom Landry; former first lady Nancy Reagan; TV commentator Phyllis George; Susan Ford Bales (the president's daughter); and actors Tommy Lee Jones and Charles Bronson. Bronson's wife, Jill Ireland, had recently died from breast cancer. Mary Kay Ash of Mary Kay cosmetics sponsored my fellowship, and it was my pleasure to escort her to the festivities and have lunch with her. Her staff gave me a personally guided tour of her production plant after the luncheon. Both my life and my mother's were moving very fast.

The International Union Against Cancer based in Lyon, France, holds a biennial international congress in even-numbered years, and the 1990 meeting was to be held in Hamburg, Germany. I had wanted to travel to Germany to search my ancestral heritage, and this conference seemed like a perfect opportunity. I would present a scientific poster abstract at the meeting, and Sally and I would get some time to tour the countryside.

Sally and I wanted very much for our children, Heather and Christiaan, to spend as much time with their grandmother as possible before her death. We reasoned that, if my sister would help care for the kids while they were with Mother, the task would not be more than Mother could tolerate. Even though we were to be gone for two weeks, we made arrangements for the children to spend only five days with Mother. A minor complication was that Dad had knee surgery just two weeks before the children's arrival, and he was using a wheelchair. He insisted that the children would be a blessing for Mother, and we agreed with some guilt. Although she was exhausted when they left, Mother later said again and again, as she became more ill, that she cherished that visit dearly. She would often laugh as she retold a particular incident or something Heather or Chris had said.

We told the children how sick Grandma was, and we hid nothing from them. They, too, have remarked that they were glad they spent time with Grandma before she died.

Knowing that time was short, Sally and I returned home at Christmas that year, and Mother pretended that all was right with the world. She baked cookies, made a large Christmas dinner, and had relatives visit the house. We could see, though, how difficult it was for her just to walk down the hallway because of her bone pain.

The following January was a busy time for me professionally, with business trips throughout Texas. Later in the month I traveled to Washington, DC, for a breast cancer education summit on Capitol Hill. The night before the event, I had dinner with Nancy Brinker, founding chairman of the Susan G. Komen Breast Cancer Foundation (now Komen for the Cure), and others who were to attend the summit. She inquired fondly about Mother, and I assured her we were doing everything we could. The next day at the conclusion of the summit, we attended an afternoon reception at the White House with Barbara Bush. *There is a lot to be done,* I told myself. *Tea at the White House is fine, but your mother is quite ill. Don't lose your focus.*

I gave an invited lecture at Duke University at the end of January (oddly, on my Mother's birthday) that focused on our clinic at M. D. Anderson for women who were at increased risk of developing breast cancer. The irony of that presentation did not escape me as I contemplated my ailing mother, as well as the anxiety that was so intrusive for her two living sisters and my own sister as they contemplated their own risk of developing breast cancer. I wondered if my preoccupation with Mother's health was detracting from my professional presentations, but feedback from colleagues assured me that I was still making sense. February brought to me the additional responsibilities of the teaching service as the attending physician at M. D. Anderson. An added complication was another trip to Washington in mid-month to discuss cancer prevention research programs in minority populations. I did not visit Mother during that trip.

It scarcely mattered, because in mid-February, I received a telephone call that would profoundly change my life and the lives of our entire family. My mother's oncologist told me with no audible emotion that she had developed acute leukemia. This is a cancer of the bone marrow and is a complication known to occur in women with breast cancer who are treated with both chemotherapy and radiation. I had blithely told patients in the past that this complication was so rare that it did not even deserve consideration. Now, one of the rare "statistics" was my own mother! The words of Major Greenwood, one of Great Britain's famous epidemiologists rang true: medical statistics are human beings with the tears wiped away. Now, however, my own tears would not go away.

This was a journey I did not want to make.

What does a physician do when the emotional pain of dealing with patients becomes too great? He retreats to the place where he can hide: his intellectual defenses. I told myself immediately that a secondary acute leukemia was not something to be dealt with in even the best of community hospitals. I called my father, who said my mother was quite ill. I explained the situation to him and said that Mother should be in a large cancer center. He knew without my saying that my preference was Johns Hopkins. I made several telephone calls to my former mentors and arranged a transfer by ambulance. Mother was admitted to the Johns Hopkins Oncology Center within twenty-four hours.

The day before she was admitted, I made a day trip to San Diego to hear a discussion about a proposal to study the drug tamoxifen for the prevention of breast cancer. I then returned to Houston to complete my duties on the inpatient hospital teaching service and took Sally to Baltimore on the first day of March so that we could see Mother. For the next four months I fought a constant struggle between my professional responsibilities and my family obligations. Should I just stop what I was doing at work and sit at my mother's side? I thought that would annoy her more than comfort her, but I did not want to appear disinterested. It was one of the most difficult conflicts of my adult life. After much inward searching, I decided to strike a balance between work and my desire to be with Mother. Were I to do it over again, I would take a leave of absence and not try to work at all. There were many times in the months preceding Mother's death that I was simply unable to do any productive work because I could not concentrate, but I was too proud to admit that her illness troubled me greatly. I could deal with it intellectually, I told myself, but I avoided wrestling with her illness emotionally until months after she died.

Hospitals are different places for doctors, families, and patients. They are especially different when the doctor stops engaging in his role as a physician and begins assuming his role as a family member. The changing roles can be disorienting, and I sensed that disorientation as I reentered Johns Hopkins for the first time after my fellowship not as a physician, but as the son of a very sick woman. The walls that seemed so familiar and reassuring before now became hostile and threatening. The staff who had been colleagues now became functionaries with critically important tasks to perform.

The weekend after Mom had been transferred to Hopkins, I flew to Baltimore to assess the situation firsthand. Our former pastor Jerry Wicklein and his wife, Pam, were very accommodating and asked that we stay in their home during our visit. They are kind, gracious people, but even their kindness could not calm me on this trip. I could see what lay ahead for my mother. Things that I had done with my patients in previous dramas many times before were about to be replayed on the same stage, but this time the tragic heroine was going to be someone I loved and cared about deeply. I knew too much of the pain, too much of the drug toxicities, too much of the long weeks in a private room with round-the-clock nurses who robbed the ill patient of all her privacy as they performed their necessary tasks. There would be constant and well-intentioned assaults upon Mother from physicians, technicians, therapists, pharmacists, and social workers, all of whom were experts and all of whom held Mother's very best interests first in their minds, but their presence would be unending and unintentionally obtrusive in their need to deliver her care. Sleepless nights, restless days, and a constant procession of strangers into our lives lay ahead.

I recalled a patient whom I had cared for in the Johns Hopkins Oncology Center during a month's rotation when I was a resident in internal medicine at Baltimore City Hospitals. She, like Mother, had been diagnosed with acute leukemia, and the intensity of the treatment had been physically and emotionally demanding for both her and her family. She was overwhelmed by the sheer number of strangers who were involved in her care. As her resident physician, I saw her more than anyone except her nurses, often visiting her bedside three or more times daily. She told me one day that she looked to me to "make sense of all this, and keep me straight about what is happening." I did the best I could, but at the end of the month, I had to move on to my next clinical assignment as all residents did every month. I felt a special bond to Mary, however, and I told her before I left on my last day that I would return to check on her progress later in the coming month. When I returned in eight or ten days, she was recovering well from her induction chemotherapy, but she had no idea who I was! I was initially astonished and a little wounded psychologically, but then I began to dissect the situation objectively. I came to understand that the emotional, physical, and spiritual trauma of the intense therapy had simply overwhelmed Mary. Her forgetting me was symptomatic of the stress we had created for her with our aggressive therapy that compounded the anxiety already induced by her life-threatening illness.

I envisioned similar, horrible crises and much more coming in my mother's future. It was like seeing two great armies poised on the battlefield before a major conflict, knowing that the coming battle was inevitable and that there was absolutely no way to avert it. The impending devastation was as vivid in my mind's eye as the incipient carnage surely must be to a commanding general before he sends many young men to certain death. I, like the general, had no choice but to stand and fight, because I knew that without an attempt to stave off this mortal enemy, Mother would be gone very, very soon.

8

Death Stops for Me

> Because I could not stop for Death, He kindly stopped for me;
> The carriage held but just ourselves And Immortality.[1]
> —Emily Dickinson

Acute leukemia is an aggressive type of cancer. It arises in the bone marrow "stem cells" that are responsible for producing the blood cells that we need to maintain vitality and homeostasis. Mother's leukemia involved her cells called granulocytes, the white blood cells that are essential to fight infection. Every day, a healthy adult makes about two pounds of these cells, and they survive in the circulation for only six to eight hours. The malignant granulocytes of acute leukemia are like juvenile delinquents from the worst street gang you have ever imagined. There are far too many of them, because the leukemic bone marrow makes them by the billions rather than by the millions, and they pass through the body's circulatory system as normal white blood cells must do. These malignant granulocytes, however, are not content to remain within the blood vessels. They invade the very tissues they are supposed to protect, causing dysfunction of lungs, liver, kidney, and brain as the result of an obstructive sludging process that arises from both their sheer numbers and their innate stickiness. They proliferate at an amazing rate, and left untreated, a patient will die within days as the berserk process robs the body of vital nutrients, diverting them all to produce ever more leukemic cells whose increasing population continues to choke the normal processes of once-healthy organs. Death comes from massive organ failure and can be accompanied by serious bleeding and infection. Treating acute leukemia is one of the greatest challenges in medical oncology. I had done it as a resident, and I had done it many times as a medical oncology fellow. I learned painfully how difficult it was for both the patient and her family, how it precipitated great physical and emotional suffering. I certainly did not want my mother to embark on the perilous journey that is acute leukemia.

The disease offered me no choice. Knowing the battle was treacherous did not make the fight any less necessary. If we did nothing, she would die in days. If we gave her the best that medicine had to offer anywhere in the world right here in the Johns Hopkins Oncology Center that I knew so well and loved so dearly, she still had only a 10–15 percent chance of a temporary recovery (called a remission). This was because she had a so-called "secondary leukemia" induced by intensive combined chemotherapy and radiation her oncologists had given her to control her recurrent breast cancer. Secondary leukemia is notoriously difficult to treat. There were moments when I was angry at her oncologists for "causing" Mother's leukemia, but I knew my anger was not rational. Her disease caused this situation, not those who were trying to save her. That did not change the fact that I knew we were in for the biggest fight of our lives, and it was Mother's life that was at stake. I could not imagine a more demanding situation for Mother, for me, or for our family.

Doctor, What if it Were Your Mother?

Jerry and Pam Wicklein said a prayer with Sally and me before we left their house for the hospital. He asked that God would give us courage and Mother, comfort. I was filled with apprehension throughout the twenty-minute drive to Johns Hopkins, and when we arrived at the oncology center, I was overcome with an unfamiliar feeling. When I was training at Hopkins, I viewed the institution as my window to the world, a springboard for marvelous career opportunities. I had met brilliant people there who taught me how to think critically about cancer, and who always challenged me to do better, to strive for excellence. They translated that perseverance and optimism into innovative therapies, and medical knowledge inched forward. I was returning now to the people I respected, and I knew intimately who they were, yet I could not delude myself into thinking they were more than I had observed firsthand.

Many times, I believe, our patients endow us with magical powers we do not possess, and yet sometimes we physicians do perform what appear to be miracles. The tragedy comes when we believe that our miracles are of our own making. Now I needed a miracle for my mother, and I knew that any miracle would have to come from God through normal people who were exceptionally trained and unusually gifted. All their abilities and dedication, though, could not guarantee a cure for Mother.

Sally and I went to the nurses' station of the leukemia service, where I quickly renewed friendships with many physicians and nurses who all told me how concerned they were about Mother and how glad they were to see me again. It had been nearly five years since I had left, and little had changed. In the hallway I found Dr. Phillip Burke, the director of the Leukemia Service, whose clinical and laboratory data I had used to write my master's thesis in epidemiology. I had spoken to him by telephone several days before to explain what I knew of the situation before Mother's transfer and to get his opinion about her treatment. Sadly, he had told me what I already knew, that secondary leukemia is very resistant to therapy, and that our chances for success were slim at best. I was at least somewhat reassured that he was willing to try the therapy he had developed during his years at Hopkins even though he could not promise success.

We went to the hematology laboratory and looked at Mom's bone marrow under the microscope. The appearance of her leukemic cells was ominous. They were large and poorly differentiated blast cells with huge nuclei, large nucleoli, and scant cytoplasm. In plain language, they were nasty- and dangerous-looking cancer cells. They were replacing her bone marrow like streams of invading barbarians, leaving little room for the normal cells of her bone marrow. She was anemic as a result of this process, but she was not yet infected or bleeding. I was thankful for that.

The therapy Phil had planned was intense, and I knew it well because I had cared for Phil's patients myself many times during my fellowship. It involved continuous intravenous infusion of a chemotherapy drug called cytosine arabinoside along with pulsed intravenous doses of another drug called daunorubicin. The therapy was so intense that we did not allow patients to eat during the therapy and recovery period so that their gastrointestinal tracts became quiescent and prevented the mucosal lining cells from undergoing their usual daily proliferation. This "bowel rest," as Phil called it, provided protection from the intense cell killing of the chemotherapy because resting cells were not affected by the chemotherapy. Dr. Burke had learned through bitter experience that if patients ate regular diets throughout the course of chemotherapy, many would suffer severe gastrointestinal bleeding and die. Nutrition was provided through intravenous feeding into a catheter placed through the skin of the chest into the large vein beneath the collarbone and directly into the vena cava. One of the medical residents called it "steak in a bottle." I was always impressed that patients never complained of hunger with this regimen even though they went without food by mouth for a minimum of four to six weeks. The progress of the leukemia and its response to therapy was monitored by weekly bone marrow aspirations that were done by a physician's assistant and read by Dr. Burke and the oncology fellows.

Phil didn't equivocate with me. He told me the treatment was going to be tough, and that the odds were against us. I already knew that. He didn't say much about this patient being my mother. I wondered why.

I left Phil and thanked him for whatever he could do, and I went to the room to speak with my parents. It was hard for me to gauge how much they knew or understood. They had received multiple explanations from many members of the care team, and I was probably being repetitious. I also knew, though, that they might have been suffering from informational and psychological overload caused by the rapidity with which things were happening, the complexity of the facts, and the severity of her illness. It was bad enough that she had battled metastatic breast cancer for years, but now the battle was being fought on two fronts. I did the best I could to keep my explanations simple, but I did not tell them everything I knew either about the breast cancer cells in her bone marrow or about the multitude of potential complications that she would face as she fought for her life.

All of my father's brothers had married nurses, and Mom and Dad were particularly close to his youngest brother, Dallas, and his wife, Diane. They had spent many summers together on the beach at Stone Harbor, New Jersey, as Dallas and Diane's children were growing up. Diane worked in a medical specialty practice just seventy miles from Baltimore in Lebanon, Pennsylvania. On most weekends throughout Mother's illness, Diane was at her side providing comfort and reassurance during the long ordeal. For this I gave her the appellation "Saint Diane." She was also there this day at the very beginning, loving us and giving support in any way she could. We all had dinner that evening at Baltimore's famous Hausner's restaurant, where our nuclear family had celebrated my undergraduate graduation from Johns Hopkins. It was a place we had previously associated with merriment. We now tried to find comfort in our presence together, but all we could do was think of Mom and her illness and that she was not with us. It was an uneasy situation, and our conversations were cautious. Diane and I knew acute leukemia all too well, but we didn't talk about what we knew. The family knew we had special knowledge, and they didn't ask us particular or directed questions. It was all just a bit too tense, and the latent anxiety imposed by Mother's illness was not typical of our usual light and carefree family interactions.

After the first few frenetic days when much is happening very quickly in the care of a patient with acute leukemia, the patient and her caregivers settle into a more structured routine. For the medical team, not much happens for the two weeks after the so-called induction therapy is given. We monitor daily laboratory work, watch for signs of bleeding or infection, and wait. Knowing this, it didn't seem reasonable for me to remain in Baltimore. Our children were in Houston, my job was in Houston, and, frankly, I was uncomfortable waiting in Baltimore. I simply knew too much about all the disastrous things that could happen, and not being there seemed to make them less likely to occur, however irrational that logic was.

As Sally and I prepared to depart for Houston, I told Dad I would call often and return soon. I kissed Mother Good-bye, and we left for the airport.

Sally and I talked earnestly about my conflict over being in Baltimore instead of Houston. She encouraged me to return to my mother whenever and however it was necessary, and I knew she was sincere. Houston was now home and a haven for me to hide in, but I did so with daily guilt, often believing that I should be with Mother.

My work in Houston (with strange irony) concentrated on women who were at risk of developing breast cancer. I had begun to publish research studies about our work. This led to a bit of national recognition for me, and two weeks after Mother was admitted to the Oncology Center, I was asked to host Linda Taira and the film crew of the CBS News show *48 Hours*, who wanted to come to my clinic and see how we were managing our patients. This seemed like an opportunity not to be missed, and I even believed that Mother would be heartened and encouraged by the recognition we had received.

I called Baltimore frequently to get updates from Dad about Mom's condition. He had moved into a facility called Rockwell House that had been built near the Oncology Center to house the families of patients who were committed to long-term stays in the hospital. This avoided the problem of securing housing in the city that was difficult to find and very expensive. Rockwell House was a block from the hospital, and it had comfortable rooms with a common kitchen area where families could congregate and eat meals together. These accommodations allowed Dad to visit Mother on a daily basis. He literally never left her side except to sleep and eat throughout the entire ten weeks she was a patient at Johns Hopkins. When I spoke with him by telephone, he would tell me of the daily routines of the nurses and physicians who were caring for Mother. Although he did not know her laboratory values with the precision of an intern or medical resident, he was able to tell me when Mom had a fever or when her platelet count was low. When there was a new problem like a fever, I called Phil Burke for more specific data.

Each week, the treatment team repeated Mom's bone marrow examination, a standard practice for the Leukemia Service. Because the primary disease with acute leukemia is in the bone marrow, examining these cells under a microscope reveals a great deal of information about the effectiveness of the therapy. In the first few weeks after the induction therapy, the bone marrow will show whether the therapy has eliminated the leukemic cells from the marrow. After that, the team waits for recovery of the normal bone marrow cells and the appearance of healthy white cells. Eventually, normal red cells and platelets appear as well. In Mom's case, the question was also one of clearing the breast cancer cells that had invaded her bone marrow.

In the first few weeks, Dad told me what I expected: the marrow was "empty" with no sign of the leukemia, the breast cancer, or much normal marrow, either. Mom was not hungry because of the intravenous hyperalimentation that provided her sufficient calories, vitamins, minerals, and other essential nutrients every day. Predictably, however, by the third week, Mom developed a fever, a sign of possible infection not at all unexpected given that she had no white blood cells to ward off invading microorganisms. I had cared for patients in these situations many times, and we had a prescribed protocol for dealing with them. We started intravenous antibiotics after obtaining appropriate cultures of blood and urine. If the fever persisted after three days, we added additional antibiotic coverage. If the temperature was still elevated after a week, we added antifungal medications. It was all very objective when I was caring for other patients, but now with Mom came nagging doubts for me. I did not question whether the team of physicians and nurses was doing everything they could for Mom. My doubt, rather, was in knowing that even with this superb care, the outcome might not be what we had hoped for.

When I spoke with Dad on the phone, I always started by asking him what the team had told him that day. He was credible at reporting the big picture, and he clued me in on the important details and new developments. I tried to be encouraging to him, and I tried to explain the mountain of data he was confronting every day.

When I was a fellow at Hopkins, Dad once joined me for morning rounds on the bone marrow transplant unit where we cared for some of the sickest patients in the entire cancer center (or in the Johns Hopkins Hospital, for that matter). Dad stayed with us for the two and a half hours that it took to make rounds on just fourteen patients, many of whom were very ill. He told me afterward that he was astonished at the amount of data that we physicians sifted through on rounds each day, and at the sheer volume of material that we processed to make our decisions.[2] We looked at vital signs and body weights, fluid intake and output, values reported from hematology, chemistry, and microbiology laboratories; X-rays, bone marrows, and reports from consultants.

We discussed our respective interpretations of the results with each other and decided what our plans should be. Sometimes we argued; often we admitted that we were not sure what course of action would be best despite the reams of data. The team always sought consensus, and we tried to present a unified plan that was developed jointly from as many as a dozen of us to the patients and their families. We also tried to be optimistic with the families as often as possible while silently harboring our own fears and festering doubts.

My emotions about Mom made working in my office on Monday morning after our return to Houston quite challenging. I couldn't concentrate, and I found my thoughts returning repeatedly to Baltimore and her. Several of my colleagues said I should be at her bedside. Most others simply offered hope and concern. My boss, Dr. Rodger Winn, director of the Community Oncology Service, said I could take as much time as I needed to be with her. I reluctantly stayed in Houston, knowing that I was avoiding participating in Mother's pain by being at work, yet her pain was still very real to me. I could not get her out of my mind, and I prayed constantly that she would not suffer. I also prayed that she would recover, because I was not ready to see her leave us at sixty-three years of age with my children only five and eight years old. I wanted Grandma to see her grandchildren grow up, and I wanted them to know her. They needed me, too, however. When I was away, it was always a burden for them, and I missed them when I traveled. Being with them and Sally was a comfort to me, but I struggled with not being with Mother every moment of that long, difficult winter and early spring. I wanted to be in Houston and Baltimore at the same time, and that was impossible.

I think my keeping busy at my job was what the psychologists call "avoidance behavior." If I manufactured "important" things to do in Houston, it eased the pain of Mom's ordeal, at least momentarily. My journal says Sally and I went to the ballet three weeks after we came home; I don't know why, because we did not attend regularly. I can only imagine that at the ballet, I did not have to contemplate Mom's illness for a few hours. I was avoiding and denying the reality at the same time.

On Palm Sunday, one month after Mother began her therapy, Sally and I took the children to Phoenix. The American Cancer Society had invited me to attend their annual Science Writers' Seminar to present the work I was doing with my high-risk patients. The society's Texas division had funded a major portion of my work in evaluating the results of the 1987 Texas Breast Screening Project, and I had published a number of research studies with colleagues using the data from the project. It seemed to Sally and me that we should accept the invitation. Dad did not object.

The seminar was arranged in panels, and each panel had a chairman. My chairman was Dr. Bernard Fisher, who at the time was the director of the National Surgical Adjuvant Breast and Bowel Project, funded by the National Cancer Institute. This research group had done some of the most important clinical trials in breast cancer during the previous twenty years, including the landmark study that proved lumpectomy (breast-conserving surgery) plus radiation was equivalent to mastectomy in controlling local recurrence of breast cancer.[3] Dr. Fisher's work ultimately saved millions of women in the United States and around the world from the trauma of undergoing mastectomy. He was one of my heroes, and here I was sitting with him explaining my work in high-risk women. I did not divulge to him that my mother had actually required treatment with mastectomy because of the size of her tumor and the involvement of multiple areas of her breast with cancer. I also did not tell him she was now at Johns Hopkins or what her diagnosis was.

He was impressed with my presentation and asked that I join him in designing and conducting a new research study that was to determine if it was possible to prevent breast cancer from occurring in high-risk women who had never had the disease.[4] I was glad I went to Phoenix, and Dr. Fisher's kindness and interest in my work eased my guilt a bit, but my thoughts were pulled continuously to my mother in Baltimore. At the seminar, CNN science correspondent Dan Rutz interviewed me about my work, and the interview appeared repeatedly on CNN over the next several weeks. The recognition was wonderful, but I still asked myself whether I was doing the right thing by not being at my mother's bedside.

By the middle of April, seven weeks after her acute leukemia diagnosis and admission to the Johns Hopkins Oncology Center, it was clear that Mother was dying. The weekly bone marrow aspirations had shown very few cells (as they always do) in the first three weeks after she received her induction therapy. By week four, her bone marrow began to repopulate with cells, but Phil Burke could not be sure what the status of her leukemia was with scant cells in the marrow. Grimly, five weeks after the induction therapy, Phil told me that Mom's marrow was showing a return of not only her leukemia cells but of her breast cancer cells as well.

What kind of cancer is this? I asked myself. *Don't those cells know that this is my mother and that she is a patient at Johns Hopkins?* The *Johns Hopkins Hospital! Those cells are not supposed to be in her bone marrow after all this aggressive therapy!* I yelled silently to myself.

I was being both emotional and irrational, and I knew it, but I did not want my mother to die. Her death was not in the plans I had scripted for my life, or hers, or her grandchildren's. I phoned my father and asked if he understood the situation. All he knew was that Mother had persistent fevers. She had been receiving continuous antibiotic and antifungal treatment for weeks. She spent most of her days sleeping, but Dad said she was still hopeful that we could find effective therapy. I told him I was coming back to Baltimore.

This was a flight I did not want to make.

The annual meeting of the Society for the Study of Breast Disease was scheduled for April in Dallas, and I was to present our data from the Texas Breast Screening Project. Dr. Fisher was expected to be in attendance. I planned to leave Dallas and fly to Baltimore on Saturday afternoon after my presentation. Sally stayed in Houston with the children. I have no recollection of what I said in my presentation at the meeting because I was consumed with thoughts of my mother. I had great apprehension about what awaited me in Baltimore. Friends and colleagues in Dallas saw my distress and urged me to go to my mother's side as quickly as possible.

As soon as my flight landed, Uncle Dallas and Aunt Diane picked me up at Baltimore Washington International Airport and drove me to the hospital. When I arrived at the oncology center, Dad was at Mom's bedside. The hospital was quiet, and spring sunlight filled her room. There were no flowers because they are not permitted due to the increased risk of infection from live plants in patients with compromised immune systems. The absence of flowers made the room look harsh and sterile. I walked to Mom's bedside and took her hand. This felt strange because we were not a family that embraced often or showed emotion openly. I was not sure how much either Mom or Dad knew about the situation or the findings on her recent bone marrow examinations, and I was certain I could not find the proper words to explain. I employed the rule I use with my patients: tell the truth, and don't evade the bad news, as difficult or as painful as it may be. This was not a time to tower over her like the knowledgeable assistant professor that I was not in this situation. Sitting in the chair next to her bed and facing her at eye level, I asked if she was aware of the bone marrow findings. She stared back blankly. Dad appeared startled. I thought he knew. I explained both the leukemia cells and the breast cancer in her bone marrow.

Mom was silent for a minute. Then she asked, "That's not good, is it?"

I wanted to scream and cry and run. I wanted to be anywhere but in that awful, stark, morosely sunny hospital room. I had let her down. We had sent her to the best hospital in the country, and they had let her down. Her fair-haired boy of promise, her companion on the great ride that is a career in medicine, had just delivered the saddest and most ominous personal news this gentle, loving, caring nurse had ever received.

All I could do was to hold her hand and tell the truth.

I told her she would stay at Hopkins until our family had decided our next course of action. I was not sure she understood. I didn't yet know if Dad grasped what I was saying, but Aunt Diane knew. I was so grateful that at least one other person in that room on that afternoon understood that I was stricken with sadness and frustration. I was about to lose my mother very soon, and I could not halt the process despite training and knowledge and professional relationships with the finest doctors in the world. The lifeguard flight that was supposed to rescue Mother was now destined to crash in a fireball.

I thought it would be wise to take Dad to Sunday services at the Arnolia United Methodist Church, where Sally and I had been members during our training, for spiritual support, to take him away from the dying process, and for some emotional relief. We drove through Homewood's Sherwood Gardens in central Baltimore in a light rain on our way back to the hospital. Dad was quiet but thankful to have gotten away from the hospital for a time.

I flew home on Tuesday after saying good-bye to Mom for what would be the last time. With each passing day, Mother's situation became more desperate. No additional treatment was going to be effective. Having done all they could at Johns Hopkins, and having no realistic hope for a cure of her leukemia with additional treatment, Dad transferred her home to St. Luke's Hospital in Bethlehem. Some of the physicians at Hopkins wanted to attempt a second induction treatment regimen, whereas the social worker advocated sending her home. Our family thought it best that she leave. She would be close to those who loved and cared for her, and Dad would be at home.

Media interest in my work continued, and the *48 Hours* show on the CBS television network that described my high-risk clinic at M. D. Anderson aired the next week. Sally and I hosted a group of friends in our home to watch the report. Dad said Mom was too ill to see it, and I don't think he was emotionally able to watch it either. It made the national recognition I received seem very hollow to me. If my mother was so ill, I asked myself, what had I really accomplished?

Thirteen days after I left her, Dad called me at my office in Houston to say that Mother had started bleeding from her intestines. This meant that the end was near, that her bone marrow could not make enough platelets to control the bleeding, and that she would die very soon. I called Sally and told her I would have to go to be with Mother immediately if I wanted to see her alive one last time. There were no flights until the next morning, so I went home to wait and mourn with Sally and our children.

Two hours after I got home, Dad called to say Mother had died with my brother, Tim, and him at her side. I told Dad my flight times for the morning, and he said he would meet me at the airport. I flew alone to the Allentown airport, and Sally and the children followed the next day.

We did things backward for Mother's memorial service. We took her body to the cemetery first and had a brief graveside service with only our family present. We then went to the church and had a service in which we celebrated her life. Hundreds of friends and family attended.

One of the most difficult church services I ever attended was on Mother's Day at First Presbyterian Church, Bethlehem, on the day after we memorialized my mother so faithfully. Some might have said that we had been to church the day before and did not need to attend again so soon. Others might have reasoned that Mother's Day was meant for celebration, and we surely had nothing to celebrate. Or did we? Mother's life and legacy were certainly a source of joy for all of us.

Doctor, What if it Were Your Mother?

Two weeks after Mother died, I had minor outpatient surgery in Houston. During my recovery at home, I wept freely over the loss we had suffered, over my disappointment that we had not been able to save her from her illnesses.

Shortly after Mother's death, I had breakfast with Marilyn Quayle, wife of the vice president, who was in Houston to receive an award from the American Association for Cancer Research. She offered me warm condolences, and I knew that her mother had also died from breast cancer years earlier. Mrs. Quayle had joined the national fight against breast cancer, making it a political focus for herself, and she and I found ourselves together repeatedly at both regional and national programs to marshal support for the cause. It was comforting to know that this prominent woman shared in my pain, and that we both knew the heartache of losing a loved one to the consequences of breast cancer.

One month after Mother died, the wives of the Houston Astros baseball team joined representatives from the Susan G. Komen Breast Cancer Foundation to present me the Tiffany & Company award for excellence in breast cancer research, teaching, and patient care. I was very grateful, but I felt undeserving, thinking that I had failed my mother and our family. I wondered what I had really accomplished. I found no joy in my work for a long time after her death. I never doubted that God was present as the pangs of loss tormented me and the visions of Mother in the oncology center haunted my dreams for many days and weeks. Yet, the joy of my salvation simply would not return. Mourning can be a slow and troubling process, even for a person of faith. I had seen this from a distance in the families of my patients. Now I was feeling it firsthand. The love of God is constant, however, and he is a very present help in times of trouble. Healing for me would come slowly over many weeks, and the beginning of the resolution of my grief would come one month after Mother died when I found myself in a jungle in Central America. I shall recount that revelation much later in the book.

---

[1] *The Complete Poems of Emily Dickinson.* Johnson, Thomas H, ed. Boston: Little, Brown & Company, 1976.

[2] Dad kept true to form on rounds, always in his pastoral mode. Rounds are challenging for the nurses, physicians, pharmacists, and support staff because there is a great deal of work to be done in a short time. Much of what occurs on rounds in a bone marrow transplant program is transfer of information. It takes great effort to make sure that everyone had the same information and the plan is clear. There is not much time to visit socially with the patients. We were making steady progress during the morning that Dad joined us, and as the medical oncology fellow conducting the rounds, I was trying to keep the pace moving so we could finish in a timely manner and get on with the rest of our work. As we left the room of a young anthropologist who had reached the recovery phase of her transplantation and was nearing the time of discharge, I noticed that Dad was nowhere to be seen. I thought perhaps that he had gone to the restroom, or that he was simply worn out from standing for nearly two hours. I excused myself from the team for a moment and walked down the hallway, retracing our steps. I found Dad engaged in a lively exchange with the young professor. He was asking about her work and her disease and her hopes for the future. I wondered silently if anyone else on our team had been so pastoral in their interest. They parted as if they were old friends after no more than five minutes of true conversation. In retrospect, the whole scene reminded me of Jesus leaving his parents in Jerusalem and going to the temple. Where else should I have expected to find the pastor than at the bedside of the patient in need, being a pastor?

[3] Fisher's work was tainted briefly with controversy related to data falsification by a Canadian surgeon in the historical surgical trial. Fisher was ultimately vindicated and the validity of his work proven and verified. This fascinating story of one of the giants of 20th century clinical research is masterfully recounted by Lisa Keränen of the University of Colorado at Denver in her intriguing narrative

Scientific Characters (Tuscaloosa: The University of Alabama Press, 2010). In my comments on the dust jacket of the book I lament that "Although some investigators will be frustrated, and some patients will be disheartened, we applaud the reality that, by God's grace, research moves on and we learn things in spite of ourselves."

[4] This trial was called the Breast Cancer Prevention Trial (BCPT), and it was a landmark in twentieth century oncology. The trial evaluated whether the hormonal drug tamoxifen could reduce the incidence of new breast cancer in women with risk factors for the disease including family history, early age at menarche, late age at first birth, never having children, or having one or more breast biopsies. Dr. Fisher asked me to serve on the Steering Committee for the trial, and I directed the largest system of clinics in the trial, enrolling more than 400 subjects through the University of Texas M. D. Anderson Cancer Center. When the trial was reported in 1998, more than 13,000 women had enrolled, and the trial demonstrated that tamoxifen reduced the incidence of new breast cancer by 49 percent in these women at increased risk. The trial was, in my opinion, the crowning achievement of Dr. Fisher's long and distinguished career. I was honored to be included as an author on the manuscript that reported the findings in the Journal of the National Cancer Institute: Fisher B, Costantino JP, Wickerham DL, et al. Tamoxifen for prevention of breast cancer: Report of the National Surgical Adjuvant Breast and Bowel Project P-1 Study. *J Natl Cancer Inst* 1998;90:1371-1388.

9

A Bulwark Never Failing

> A mighty fortress is our God, a bulwark never failing; Our helper He amid the flood of mortal ills prevailing. For still our ancient foe doth seek to work us woe; His craft and power are great, and armed with cruel hate, On earth is not his equal.[1]
> —Martin Luther, *Ein' feste berg ist unser Gott* ("A Mighty Fortress Is Our God")

I will propose throughout the rest of this book that we can greatly improve much of what is wrong in our health care system, help patients and their families make better choices at the end of their lives, and reduce the cost of our care simply by improving how doctors and patients discuss and weigh the many choices that confront us as we die. What follows here is my most cherished illustration about optimal communication between a doctor, a patient, and her family who were once strangers but who walked together along a challenging path to her eventual and peaceful death.

One of the functions of a comprehensive cancer center is to provide second opinions to patients who have received a diagnosis of cancer at another institution. These patients and their families are understandably anxious to know that the information provided to them by their physicians is accurate and reflects the most current and widely accepted recommendations for diagnosis and therapy. Rarely, a patient and her family hope to have the cancer diagnosis reversed, and this can happen. I can remember only two patients who had a diagnosis altered from malignant to benign through consultation, and for them, our treatment recommendation was, of course, radically different from the proposed treatment for the presumed malignancy. But these two cases are rare clinical exceptions. After fifty years of formalized training for medical oncologists, the field is now populated with many expert clinicians who can reliably diagnose cancer and make prudent treatment recommendations. This training and expertise is also available throughout Europe, and our European colleagues have contributed extensively to our knowledge of the diagnosis and treatment of cancer.

Nevertheless, there are patients and their families who, in the face of the diagnosis of a serious illness, insist on making lengthy pilgrimages beyond perfectly adequate medical care to remote academic centers where they believe unique and more effective therapy is available. With the dissemination of academic and clinical expertise on both sides of the Atlantic, and with the rapid proliferation of medical journals and meetings, there is often only reassurance to be given during such a consultations. I do not want to minimize, however, the importance of reassurance; indeed, I dispense a great deal of it.

For the consulting physician in an academic cancer center, many patients come for a lengthy and comprehensive initial evaluation and then return to their treating physician without coming back again for additional consultation. This fact made it difficult for me to establish the usual type of physician-patient bond in many of the clinical interactions that confronted me as an academic physician. Occasionally, however, a patient appeared who asked more or needed more or demanded more from me, and the effect of these patients on me endured well beyond the time of our initial encounter. Hilda Muller was such a patient.

Hilda and I met through the Community Oncology Referral Service at M. D. Anderson. Her breast cancer was diagnosed at her home in Germany. The primary tumor was moderately sized at two centimeters, and none of fifteen axillary lymph nodes was found to be involved with metastatic tumor during her modified radical mastectomy. Her prognosis was excellent as assessed by all the usual clinical parameters. She underwent standard adjuvant chemotherapy (therapy added to surgery to improve the chance of survival and to decrease the chance of relapse), and she remained well for the next three years, staying quite active as the mother of two teenagers and the wife of a successful small-business man.

Just over three years after her mastectomy, however, one of the tumor markers (a protein assayed in blood) began to rise. A small growth appeared in the space above her right clavicle, and her surgeon performed a diagnostic biopsy that confirmed the presence of recurrent breast cancer. She was followed conservatively and appropriately for six months when both ovaries were removed surgically. She was fifty-two years old. There is a growing body of medical literature that shows a benefit from removing the ovaries in some breast cancer patients, and the procedure stabilized the situation for Hilda for the next six months. Soon, though, the mass above her right collarbone reappeared, and this time the surgeon could not completely remove the growth. A partial resection was possible, and examination of this tissue confirmed persistent, recurrent breast cancer with the presence of both estrogen and progesterone receptors in the tumor.

The presence of estrogen and progesterone proteins is a hopeful sign in that it portends a more favorable prognosis and greater responsiveness to both chemical and hormonal therapies. Recognizing these facts, her physicians in Germany began treatment with the hormone tamoxifen immediately after learning these findings. Unfortunately, after six weeks of hormonal therapy, her tumor markers began to rise again, and her chemotherapy was restarted. The progression of her tumor caused great and understandable concern in Hilda's husband, Rolf, who then initiated a search for answers about Hilda's breast cancer on both sides of the Atlantic.

They visited the cancer centers at Harvard University and the Mayo Clinic before they arrived in Houston. She had seen some of the finest oncologists in the world and had received what amounted to variations on the same theme: additional chemotherapy was necessary, and it could be either the chemotherapy she received before or two drugs identical to those she had received in the past plus one new drug. There were mixed thoughts about the usefulness of the hormonal therapy. The Mullers wanted to know what I thought as a young assistant professor.

I spent twenty minutes reviewing the records Hilda brought with her and another thirty taking a confirmatory history with Rolf serving as the interpreter. (We have since abandoned the process of using family members as interpreters in these situations for a number of complex medical, ethical, and legal reasons, but during all my interactions with Hilda, Rolf performed admirably.) He asked that I speak slowly, saying that his English was not so good. In fact, his English was impeccable, and he kept fastidious notes about her care along with recording in minute detail what he was told by their many consultants.

A true German, I thought to myself with a personal pride that recalled the meticulous precision of my Pennsylvania Dutch (i.e., *Deutch*) relatives, some of whom could even be called persnickety. This trait is hardly unique to those of us of Germanic descent, though. I once cared for the wife of a chemical engineer who was as American as apple pie. She had acute leukemia and was quite ill. He met us at the door of her room each day, clipboard in hand, to recount the daily laboratory work with greater detail and precision than even my finest medical resident could muster. He even graphed her daily progress! Our team members constantly feared that he would know something about the patient that we did not, but this embarrassment never occurred. We eventually learned that his clipboard was the engineer's best mechanism for coping with the extreme stress that his wife's illness caused him, and we were not about to take away an effective coping strategy.

So it was with Rolf: he was exhaustingly thorough with his questions, remembered everything I said, and completed a sort of comparative oncologic exercise as he weighed my recommendations with those of the other consultants. The process was, surprisingly, neither irritating nor exhausting, and I was impressed by the care and concern this man showed for his wife. I spent nearly an hour answering his questions as Hilda listened attentively. She spoke little English but understood a great deal, as I would eventually learn. In the beginning I was not sure that Rolf accepted what I was saying. He seemed hesitant and doubtful, almost suspicious. He would then surprise me by saying that the other consultants had given the same advice or made the same recommendation.

As the hour passed, I began to develop a unique fondness for this couple, who were unlike any other people I had seen and examined. We developed a rapport so quickly that at the end of our time together, Rolf produced a manila envelope from which he took a five-by-seven-inch photograph of his neighbor (who was also his mayor) chipping away at the Berlin Wall. He presented me with the picture along with a small piece of the wall. He then offered that if I were ever in Germany, I should visit Hilda and him. Ironically, I was planning to be in Hamburg in just four months for the biennial meeting of the UICC, The Union for International Cancer Control (previously named the International Union Against Cancer, or UICC from the French *Union Internationale Contre le Cancer*). The organisation holds a biennial meeting which rotates among cities of the world to attract practicing physicians, public health officials, non-governmental organizations, and medical researchers to share information and promote good will. The Mullers' home in Aurich was only seventy miles away. I did not mention the meeting at the time, but I filed away the possibility that I would visit them later that year.

As Sally and I made our plans for the trip to Europe for the UICC meeting, we explored the possibility of a stop in Aurich. We reasoned that a rail pass would be an excellent way to travel from our arrival city of Paris through the German countryside to Hamburg. The pass included a boat excursion on the Rhine from Mainz to Cologne, so it seemed perfect to include a short trip from Hamburg to Aurich. With some self-consciousness, I wrote to the Mullers and asked whether they really meant to invite the American oncologist to their home, and Rolf quickly replied in the affirmative.

After settling in Hamburg for a few days to initiate the medical meeting, we took the train to Bremen on Friday evening to meet Rolf at the *bahnhof*. We arranged by telephone for our simultaneous arrivals, and he found us within minutes of our stepping from the *Bundesbahn* coach.

"*Gutten naben, Herr* Muller!" I hammed as we approached with outstretched hands.

"*Gutten naben, Herr Doktor*!" welcomed Rolf in the last German he would address toward us for the weekend. I introduced Sally, and we got in the waiting car.

There was a forty-minute drive in front of us, and I wondered if it would be awkward. Rolf had never met Sally, and he and I had had only the single encounter in the clinic. To our delight, he was the perfect tour guide. He narrated the entire trip through beautiful and pastoral German farmland. I felt strangely at home.

As we approached Aurich, Rolf apologized that we would have to sleep in "the world's smallest room" in their house, a house that turned out to be warm and inviting. Hilda greeted us eagerly and introduced us to their children, who both spoke perfect English. I explained to the Mullers that it was a constant embarrassment to me as an American that I spoke only one other language (French) and did not do that well. They did not seem to mind.

Hilda produced a spectacular meal for us that began with a huge plate of cold fish that I mistakenly believed was the entire meal. I gorged myself on herring and eel, a particular delicacy of northern Germany. When I announced that I enjoyed the eel, Rolf declared that I could not have eaten any, because there was no eel skin on my plate.

"No eel skin!" he observed.

"I ate the eel skin," I announced sheepishly.

There was momentary silence and our hosts exchanged furtive glances around the table.

"You will need a doctor, *Herr Doktor!*" Rolf declared before breaking into raucous laughter with his family. For a moment, Sally and I did not know what to think, but the predicted ill effects never arrived, and we laughed with our hosts as we enjoyed a lovely veal dinner well into the evening.

After dinner we spoke with the Muller children about their schooling and about Conrad's imminent required service in the German army. Near eleven o'clock, when Sally and I were very much thinking about turning in for the night, Rolf told us that the town was having a festival and that there were grand happenings in the city square that would last well into the night.

"Do you want to go to the festival?" he wanted to know.

When we hesitated because of the late hour, he urged me to join him in just *"ein bier."* Ah, that wonderful, smooth, refreshing German beer. Why not? After the beer, it was off to the festival.

Hilda did well with the burden of preparing dinner for six and the late-night walk through the town square, but by the next morning, she was exhausted. Rolf had an elaborate touring itinerary planned through the beautiful countryside that is Friesland, Aurich's home district in the northwest corner of Germany in the same low country that becomes the Netherlands to the west. To my surprise, this part of Germany, in stark contrast to the Rhine valley, is filled with dikes and moors, windmills and bogs that give it a quaint charm visible in each building and home and in the eyes of all the citizens. With Hilda resting comfortably at home, Rolf and Sally and I spent the morning exploring the countryside and its water castles, its windmills, and its uncommonly plain church exteriors that hide some of the most spectacular baroque interiors and magnificent pipe organs in all the world.

We stopped at the family business, Supermarket Muller, for a quick tour and retrieval of coffee and jam souvenirs. Slowly, we were learning who these special people were.

After a morning of touring, we met Hilda at the Mullers' small sailing boat on the East Frisian Islands in the North Sea just west of Helgoland Bay where the Weser River drains Lower Saxony, flowing past Bremen. Here Rolf and Hilda had spent many summers with the children. They had sailed the twenty-three-foot craft to many ports of the Mediterranean Sea over the years as their children grew up. It was immediately clear that the boat was special to them, and they took care in ensuring that we would see it and know what an important role it had played in their lives. We ate lunch on the boat amid tales of good weather and bad, of exciting ports of call, and of happier times.

Back at their home, Sally and Hilda somehow conversed for three hours during the afternoon as they prepared dinner, Sally speaking no German and Hilda no English! Sally learned that Hilda's father had been killed in World War II, and Sally shared that her father, like Rolf, was a small-business man. Rolf and I shared pleasant talk of our respective views of medicine and business over bottles of fine German beer as he grilled our steaks on the patio. These were amiable and gracious people opening their home to us as if we were family.

There came a time in our conversation when Rolf asked very naturally about my extended family. Sally and I had told Hilda and him about our children from the moment we met. Now he was asking about my parents, and my brother and sister. It is true that we had crossed the line that usually separates doctor from patient when I made this transoceanic house call and accepted the warm German hospitality of this pleasant couple. Initially, my inclination was to avoid the issue completely, but it was obvious that would have been impolite. I personally did not object to revealing details of my mother's breast cancer, but I feared it would put the Mullers in the awkward position of wanting to express concern over her illness while needing to receive expert consultation from me.

We deceive ourselves in the medical profession if we believe that complete personal anonymity from our patients is desirable. Many of them want to know about our families and our personal lives. They want to know that we are human beings, and they want to know about the people we care for outside our professional lives. That is not to say that physicians do not need privacy, and it is certainly true that there are some facts about my personal life that I would not want displayed in the public square. As I moved closer to the Mullers, I reflected on the closeness I had encountered with other patients and families. I wondered if I had lessened the quality of my therapeutic interventions with my patient and her husband by telling them that my mother was dying. Did the revelation of this knowledge somehow impair my objectivity? I reasoned that if I was crippled by my emotions arising out of the circumstances in my family life, I would not serve the needs of my patients through silence and repression. I have come to believe that I can meet some of the needs of my patients through their knowing that I am suffering in ways that are like their own suffering.

It is also clear to me that empathetic suffering alone is not enough. I do not diminish the intensity or the pain of my patient's suffering simply by acknowledging that I, too, suffer. My patients want me to bring technical competence and clinical skill to the bedside. To say to my patient merely that I have suffered in the same way she is suffering offers little or no comfort. Some patients may even regard such statements as crass and uncaring. It is also true that if his own emotional tension, strife, and grief become overwhelming, the physician should remove himself from clinical situations in which he is expected to be objective and possess the ability to think clearly without compromise. No one deserves an impaired physician. If a physician in the midst of a therapeutic relationship with a patient were to unburden his personal concerns in the hope of receiving therapeutic support from the patient, such behavior would be considered overtly inappropriate. Expressing human concern for one's own family member is not impairment, however, and sharing a situation of illness in a physician's family briefly with a patient is an opportunity to relate emotionally with a patient. This bonding with the patient enhances the therapeutic relationship by instilling trust through personal authenticity.

Rolf and Hilda expressed their concern for my mother openly and warmly, and they offered their best wishes for her recovery and for my peace of mind. Our stay was brief at just over twenty-four hours, and Sally and I were both reluctant to leave after our second dinner with the Mullers. It did not seem reasonable to stay longer, though, because our continued visit was a physical burden for Hilda. We parted eager for more time together, which is the way it should have been. Sally and I promised Rolf we would see Hilda and him again soon on their next visit to M. D. Anderson.

Rolf and Hilda Visit Houston

Just seven months later, Rolf called and said he wanted Hilda to come for an annual checkup so that I could review her records from Germany and make any suggestions to alter her care. She was receiving monthly intravenous injections of a medication to control her bone metastases, and I offered to give it to her at our clinic. We enjoyed having them in our home, and we arranged dinners with our friends so we could share these lovely Germans of whom we were becoming so very fond.

Hilda felt well but tired easily. Fortunately, medication was keeping her bone pain under control. On the third day of their visit, the ever-adventuresome Rolf announced to me that he wanted to take a trip to Mexico. He wanted to know if I thought Hilda could tolerate the journey. With her bone pain under control, I did not see why not until he told me that he wanted to drive from Houston to Mexico City! That distance is more than 800 miles, and I had heard tales of road bandits who forced motorists off the highway at night to commit armed robbery or worse crimes. I also had doubts about any of the major car-rental companies allowing a foreigner to drive a rented car to Mexico.

Rolf would not be deterred. I thought initially that he was being somewhat reckless, taking his sick wife on such a long drive. I thought he was denying the severity of her illness, pretending that she was well, trying to recapture happy, earlier days when they traveled with their children through Europe. I slowly came to understand, however, that this trip had another purpose: it was probably their last because her disease was progressing, and I couldn't stop it.

I drove him around Houston and checked with several car-rental agencies. All declined to make the rental. Rolf, however, being a world traveler and a seasoned adventurer, suggested we inquire at a car dealership. I thought it was a ridiculous idea. The thought had not occurred to me that they would rent cars, especially to travel out of the country. To my amazement and Rolf's delight, the first dealer we asked agreed and even offered very favorable weekly rates.

The Mullers were gone two weeks. They sent us a postcard from Mexico City indicating they were enjoying their trip. I was simply relieved to know they had arrived, and I hoped quietly to myself that they would return safely to Houston with Hilda still free of symptoms. When they did arrive safely, they both appeared rested, even after such an arduous journey. Privately, though, Rolf admitted to me that he would not make the trip again because the road conditions were primitive at times. Although he never admitted it to me, I also believe he was concerned about Hilda's safety and well-being during the entire trip. He must have asked himself often what he would do if she were to get ill out in the Mexican desert hundreds of miles from adequate medical care. I told him that I was so glad he had not had to confront that question.

Sadly, Rolf came to the realization on that trip that Hilda was dying. I have never devised a satisfactory clinical or physiological explanation for myself that unravels the complexities of how patients know when the end is approaching, but I have no doubts that they do. We can plot it clinically by simply graphing what we call performance status, a composite summary of how much patients care for themselves and what their usual daily activities are. When these things start to falter, when the patient has less energy, when they spend more time in bed each day even while at home, the end is approaching. This measure of disease progression turns out to be as useful as any laboratory or X-ray test we can perform, and patients and their families know, in my experience, that their performance status is declining even before we point it out to them during clinical visits.

As we had learned at their home in Aurich, Hilda was a gracious and generous person even in the face of her debilitating illness. Most remarkable, her generosity did not remain at home. She enjoyed our children a great deal, and she brought them a beautiful doll and a gangly marionette from Mexico. She laughed heartily with them and communicated using very little English. Our daughter, Heather (a second grader at the time), wanted to share with Hilda in a special way and thank her for the doll. She had just completed an assignment in school in which she was asked to write about a hero she knew. Heather wrote this:

> My dad is a hero because he is doing research on cancer. He helps sick people get well. My dad teaches other doctors how to prevent cancer. Last summer he went to Europe for a meeting. Also he takes care of patients from foreign countrys [sic]. My dad is a hero because he is a doctor.
>
> Heather

That little passage filled me with both tears and pride, and Hilda and Rolf thought it was special because the trip Heather referred to was the one that took Sally and me to the their home. Rolf agreed that Heather's daddy was a hero, and I was embarrassed.

Rolf often asked me about my mother, and during their visit, Mother was dying from the recurrence of her breast cancer and the leukemia induced by her treatment. He knew how sick she was, because I could not conceal the truth of my concerns in the dispassionate terms of the clinician that I used to describe her medical condition. Rolf and I had first shared my concerns for Mother at his grill on the patio in Aurich as he made our evening supper. He was cautious and I was careful to be sparing of medical details, because I did not want him to conclude that any of the events of my mother's clinical course would necessarily be repeated in Hilda's illness. He seemed to understand and accept my vagueness when I spoke about Mother. I wondered if Rolf knew I was trying to protect him, and I wondered if I was doing as much as I could to support him emotionally.

Mother died just two months after the Mullers' visit, and I told Rolf the news in one of our frequent phone calls during which he updated me about Hilda's condition. He was genuinely sorry for my loss, and it troubled me to know that he was seeing his future in my mother's death. I wished he did not have to know, but we were friends now, and I had to tell him. It was no different, I believed, than if I had been a friend he had met in the clinic who had just lost his mother. The difference was that I was one of Hilda's doctors, and I was closer to Rolf than to the husband of any of my previous patients. My escape, my psychological alibi, was that Hilda was becoming progressively debilitated, and the Mullers would not be able to travel from Germany to Houston again. Hilda was getting excellent care at home, and the telephone calls from Rolf were reassuring in that he said she was quite comfortable.

As Hilda's illness progressed, Rolf's telephone calls stopped, but not the communication. Late in November, just eight months after their trip to Mexico, Rolf sent me a copy of a letter that Hilda had written and asked him to send to her closest friends. She wrote the letter during her prolonged final stay at what she called a "clinic" in Mischwald, Germany, that we would probably call a hospice:

November 12, 3 p.m.

I am sitting in the sun and I am enjoying the last sunshine in Meschede. I got here 14 days ago. I recuperated somewhat and I am feeling at ease. The matter in Brussels [where she had gone for additional consultations] with all the treatments was very hard on me. In between I often went to the clinic in Sauerland and also for a short visit to Crete. I enjoyed the vacation very much, but things on Crete were a bit difficult for me. But Rolf always helped me a lot, and therefore I could enjoy many things. The weather was also beautiful, but I did have to go back to Meschede because of all the pains. I was hardly at home. Right now I feel a lot better. I can move again. Of course I can't totally do it without pain medication, but I try to take less. "Build-up" baths are like small miracles for me. Recently, I can also eat again. Therefore, I feel stronger, but not in regard to weight; that I did not maintain. But for my bones, it is not too bad.

On Monday, I started a new chemotherapy. I will wait and see what it will bring. On Thursday, I will go to the clinic in Dortmund. There they will make CT scans of my head. Then they will decide whether or not to give radiotherapy. I will see what can be done.

I am very thankful to be able to be in this clinic. It is just beautiful here! The room is nice and light, and it doesn't look like a hospital room. We can choose the food from the Bistro. The nurses and the doctors are pleasant and not arrogant. I can talk to all of them, and that applies to the rest of the clinic staff as well. I have the feeling that everything is done just for me. I can also talk to the other patients easily; unfortunately, one cannot always do that with healthy people. Healthy people often become sad when talking about such things. This is a shame because slowly I am getting used to this, and I am trying to live with it. Also, I try to live well and happy, if it is possible.

But now, enough about my illness. This house is situated beautifully in Mischwald. The coloring of the leaves is beautiful now. Rolf has made some fantastic slides of it. We have heard a nice lecture on it, and Rolf showed slides from Crete and Stromboli. In between I am often in the "ergo" room [the ergonomic or exercise room]. There everyone works diligently. But many times we drink tea and eat cake there. Many pretty things are hand-crafted there like pottery, silk work, jewelry and many other things. Three ladies are here that help the sick. They are wonderful, great, educated people, with great ideas that distract the patients and make them happy. I ask myself how men and women accept these things and how very ill people can withstand them.

I, myself am now a bit lazy. I am not doing a lot. Before Christmas, I decided to do less. Everything has been too much for me. I hope that my many friends and acquaintances are understanding. I am not so strong anymore, I do not have the strength. I try to do as much as possible for myself, and I think this is good. Therefore, I am writing this round-letter to all my dear friends and will also write each one a few lines. I hope this will be fine. At least I managed to write some.

Many regards, Your Hilda

Hilda died peacefully at Mischwald just six weeks after she wrote the letter to her friends. Rolf wrote to us after she died and enclosed a number of items that were related to Hilda's last days. On the front of Hilda's memorial service program were the words to Reinhold Neibur's "Serenity Prayer" in German:

"Grant me the strength to endure the things I cannot change, Courage to change the things I can, And wisdom to know the difference."

Rolf also enclosed the family Christmas letter written just weeks before Hilda died. He wrote in the letter, "Friends are flowers in the garden of life." He related that the last two years of her life had been especially hard for Hilda, including the death of her own mother just four months before she died. He said he and Hilda wanted to see all their friends again because life was so short. He said their daughter was missing her mother very often, and that now he knew that mothers are the biggest flowers in the garden of life. He wrote that it was hard to believe how much mothers work for the family. He spoke of their trip to the United States and Mexico and to Crete. He kindly said that their friends in America tried to help them. He revealed that he had hoped he and the children could celebrate Christmas with Hilda at home or in the clinic at Meschede in Sauerland. He finished by saying that they were praying for the health of the mothers of the recipients of the letter (although mine had died seven months earlier), and that he hoped we would do the same for them. He signed it, "Thank you, Rolf."

Rolf was seeking miracles in the months before Hilda died. He wanted to find someone somewhere who had a treatment that could arrest her cancer. I repeatedly and reassuringly told him that he had identified the best care the world had to offer for breast cancer, and that the best it could do was keep the cancer in check for a while. It could be controlled but not cured. He often telephoned me from Germany to update me on Hilda's progress and to ask if by any chance, there was some new therapy that Hilda should receive that perhaps he had not yet identified. I assured him there was not. During one lengthy and somewhat repetitive conversation in which we covered clinical information we had been over many times previously, I said to Rolf that all I had to offer at this point was prayer, because our treatments were surely futile. There was a pensive "Hmm" at the other end of the phone, and I was not sure that I had been helpful. I was trying to avoid having this very concerned husband transport his increasingly sick wife from clinic to clinic around the world, looking for miracles in medicines that did not exist. I could not tell from his response whether he comprehended what I was saying.

---

[1] *Ein' feste berg ist unser Gott* (A Mighty Fortress Is Our God), Martin Luther 1529, The United Methodist Hymnal. Nashville: The United Methodist Publishing House, 1989, No. 110

10
Faith, Reason, and Suffering with Technology

> The most beautiful people we have known are those who have known defeat, known suffering, known struggle, known loss, and have found their way out of the depths.[1]
> —Elisabeth Kübler-Ross

The costs of caring for patients with cancer are divided into three important groups: 24 percent of cancer care costs are related to drugs, 54 percent to hospital care, and 22 percent to physician charges. Experts tell us that these costs can be reduced.[2] One of the most important ways is to reduce the amount we spend for care in the last month of life. One quarter of Medicare costs occur in the last year of life, and 10 percent of the total Medicare budget is spent on care in the last month of life. As we have seen earlier, among patients older than sixty-five years, fewer than one in three die in hospital, and only half use hospice services.

I believe that faith is the only solution to our predicament of not being able to assure our futures with the promises of technology. By that I mean the faith in the assurance that when you have done all you can do, there is nothing more to be done. We cannot assure our futures by convincing ourselves with technology that we are well today. Doubtless we can avert much pain and suffering for a time by adhering to reasonable standards of preventive health care. Even screening, healthful lifestyles, and vaccines fail to prevent all illness, however. We simply cannot ask medical technology to assure our futures. One of the strangest things I hear my patients saying is that they can't understand how a healthy person can suddenly become ill. The underlying assumption is that if you are well, you will continue to be well. In a moment of sheer philosophical insight a mechanic once told me, "Doc, it works until it breaks!" For most of us, we are well for a time—often a very long time—but it cannot be true forever and for everyone.[3] Today's events do not predict those of the future,[4] and it is simply not possible to assure that I will be well tomorrow by doing tests today that declare that I am well. Nor can healthful living make such guarantees.

Confident assurances about the future come only through faith in God. Such reassurances are not made more firm by particular ritualistic practices or sacrifices, but simply by the confident acceptance that the future is part of eternity controlled by a being who is far greater than our small ability to comprehend the complexities of things unseen. We cannot see the future by purchasing unnecessary medical technology that falsely convinces us we will be well tomorrow. We know that we will ultimately not be well, that we will encounter the limits of our sojourn in this life. Grace and peace come to those who recognize that faith alone overcomes fear and doubt. Faith liberates us from material enslavement to technology and determinism and from their false, temporary soothing of our anxieties about our uncertain futures.

If we medical practitioners are to recapture the fullness of our profession, we must do so by returning to a recognition that our patients have profound spiritual dimensions that hold great comfort for them.[5] Their spiritual side will not make them physically whole all of the time or permanently, but it will capture solutions that cannot be addressed by technology alone.

A Christian View

I would not want to imply that embracing faith and finding assurances about the future through belief is either simple or trivial. It is certainly not a place that is arrived at through ignorance or misinformation. I myself feel that it is very difficult to accept the Christian admonition that I must lose my life in order to find it, because I am simply too self-conscious and too competitive to allow this to happen.[6] This is what I have been trained to be. Competitiveness is what our educations and our society prepare us to embrace. This competitiveness impedes our attempts to understand suffering and pain, because we defiantly and stubbornly will not accept a burden without either a tacit, immediately visible reward or, at least, the promise of a future reward. We are eager to accept falsehoods as truth in the absence of substantiating evidence, and we let our minds be deceived if it brings us benefit.[7] We are quite willing, for example, to accept without questioning the cheap grace of the television evangelist, or the false hope of Easter without the cross. Our scientific, rational minds demand proof of the existence of God before we will yield to faith, but this is no faith at all that first demands a proof.[8] This search to explain all things through our rational minds is, perhaps, the ultimate human folly. Our obstinate disbelief may be the one unpardonable sin.[9]

Faith is a gift of the spirit, and it leads us to believe without seeing. When I am truly contemplative, I conclude that the universe is not an accident, and that we are not a random product of changeable, physical laws programmed for eventual extinction. Physicist and 1997 Nobel Laureate William Phillips of the University of Maryland told me at a meeting on science and religion at Harvard University several years ago that his agnostic scientific colleagues don't believe in God because they don't know enough physics. I took that to mean that a thorough understanding of the laws of the physical universe leads a discerning scientist to conclude that God is in the details. Dr. Phillips is a practicing Methodist, and he shared a video of his singing in his church choir during his address at Harvard to the shock, surprise, and delight of the audience.

When I studied chemistry in college, I was impressed with the order in the creation unveiled by the thermodynamicists in the eighteenth and nineteenth centuries. In one well-written college text, the three laws of thermodynamics were paraphrased with a gambling idiom: the first law states that the odds are against you; the second, that you cannot win; and the third that you cannot get out of the game. Two centuries of physical inquiry have, in fact, told us that human life is a very unlikely event. Many laws of the universe say that the whole creation should be flying apart rather than somehow miraculously holding together.

I remain faithful, therefore, not because I am ignorant of the laws of the physical universe, but rather because my knowledge of the physical universe reassures me that there exists a Divine Overseer to make the machine run.[10] This is the strongest scientific argument I can make for the existence of God—although none is required—in that it suggests that the laws that govern the physical universe may, indeed, adequately describe the reasons for an ordered, structured physical world. Experience tells us with certainty, however, that physical laws cannot and will not explain why we are allowed to suffer by a God who loves us. Explanations that appeal to inherent sinfulness (i.e., Original Sin) also appear desperately inadequate to me, especially in cases of apparently innocent suffering—such as that experienced by ill, newborn infants—unless we accept that the human race is born into sinfulness, that none of us is ever truly innocent.

Both the ancients and the scientists of the Enlightenment pondered the creation with wonderment. All of the physical universe pointed them to a creator, but we have become so introspective that we are blind to external realities learned centuries ago by even the greatest scientists:

> The true God is eternal and infinite, Omnipotent and omniscient. That is, his duration reaches from eternity to eternity; His presence, from infinity to infinity.[11]

Woefully, our materialism is so egotistical that we often cannot see the material world beyond ourselves, except for that which we perceive would satisfy our physical needs. In our intense introspection, selfishness, and scientific objectivity, we deny all the wonder, all the beauty, and all the mystery of creation. We have thereby made the creation threatening, but the creation that threatens is our creation, not God's. It is in this context that our understanding of and our approach to the suffering in our world must be evaluated.

Where Is God When We Suffer?

It is central to my Christian belief that God is eternal and infinite, the very God of very gods, the great "I Am."[12] He created the universe as part of his divine plan, portions of which are knowable to me. There are many other parts that God, in his providence, has chosen to reveal to me only in stages or not at all. Indeed, there are qualifications to the realities of his universe.

First, there are times when God reveals himself to us suddenly and dramatically, as in the birth, life, death, and resurrection of Jesus Christ. Second, there are periods of time, some inexplicably protracted, when God's revelation appears absent, such as during the Holocaust of the twentieth century or during the theologically and prophetically silent four centuries of the inter-Testament period. Third, it is probable that God's apparent absences from the human condition, his seeming indifference to human suffering, are a result of humanity's willfully turning away from the divine reality (or falsely presuming to know what the divine reality is without its being first revealed) rather than a result of his willful withdrawal.[13] Last, I believe that it is unmistakably within God's providence to send punishment and judgment should this be his will. Without this possibility God could not for me remain God (i.e., he must be omnipotent). This fact is, I believe, the proximate cause of our turning away from God. The fact that God could choose to punish us is a reality that is too painful, too difficult for us to comprehend. Why should children not be allowed to do as they please? What sort of a loving parent, we self-indulgent materialists ask, would rebuke or chastise a child?

The nonbeliever struggles to find an adequate explanation for the problem of suffering, especially when it occurs without a supposedly proper antecedent. "Why do the wicked prosper and the righteous perish?" we ask.[14] Recent explanations have cast human suffering as a random, haphazard occurrence that is no respecter of persons,[15] but these explanations beg the question. Why should suffering occur randomly? Is not this type of poorly begotten affliction meted out even more cruelly than punishment for specific offenses? Random suffering is a natural device in a deterministic, mechanistic world that is at once both hostile and impersonal. I must acknowledge, however, that it is difficult to justify punishment while, at the same time, accepting the notion of the compassionate creator.

The question "Why do we suffer and die?" is a terribly difficult quandary for us because we begin with a false premise, that we deserve neither suffering nor death. If we are "good people," as Kushner argued, why should bad things happen to us?[16] At the heart of this question is an egotistical, world-denying presumption that we are unworthy of suffering and condemnation. We *are* good, we argue. We want only the best for our families and ourselves, and we work hard to achieve those things. We are diligent in our occupations, faithful in our relationships, and engaged in our communities. We participate in civic activities, volunteer in our schools, serve on church, mosque or synagogue committees, and make donations to charities. In our own eyes, we have worked hard for our children and our spouses, and we deserve the best with no possibility of suffering.

Or do we? When I honestly examine my motives for some of my kindnesses and generosity, I sadly discover that I am often motivated not by altruism or love for my family, friends, and community but rather by my selfish desires for recognition and adulation. Martin Luther said it with elegant simplicity: "Every good work is sin."[17] Regrettably, I don't love others as much as I love myself, my motives are sometimes corrupt, and, rarely, I even wish ardently for the destruction of those who impede my personal, selfish goals! When I competed brutally with my colleagues for academic recognition and advancement, I proclaimed that I was working hard in the interest of my family. When I donate time and money publicly to worthy causes, I say that I am helping the community address its problems, to make our world a better place. When I volunteer at work or church, I say I am being generous and gracious in the interest of my colleagues or my congregation.

Am I? When I send my children to school, I say it is for them, but how much of it is for me? The school provides child care while I selfishly pursue my own interests instead of attending to the needs of my children. Of course we want professional teachers to instruct our children, and of course, we want them to have the social benefits of being schooled with other children. I am speaking here, though, of my motives. I want all those things for my children, but don't I also want my child to be successful, as judged by contemporary standards? Don't I want my child to do better than his peers, to attend the best university, to get the best, most lucrative job, to live in the most desirable community? Of course I do, but what is my motive? It is certainly because I love my children, as other parents love their children, but there is a dark motive behind this and most other good wishes we have for others. I want my children to be successful so that they won't be a burden for me! No parent wants a child to be a burden. If we were truly good, it wouldn't matter. We would be willing to say that we would shoulder any burden, pay any price, carry any load for those we love, but that kind of human devotion is so rare that we all notice it when it occurs, and we grant civic honors to those who show it.

We want our families, loved ones, friends, and associates to be well, successful, and happy, to be sure, but much of our well-wishing is selfishly motivated. When our families are well and happy, our burdens are light. When they suffer, we suffer, and we are required to carry burdens that we do not willingly want to shoulder. If my parent is suffering chronically from illness, infirmity, or disability, it is certainly a human tragedy, but my mind is not so concerned by the existential, metaphysical nuances and consequences of human tragedy. I simply want my burden to be light. I was relieved, for example, when my father's final illness, cancer of the pancreas, was blissfully brief, and he died peacefully and quietly in a few weeks rather than after a long, protracted illness at age eighty-six. It was easier for all of us that way.

Few of us ever consider suffering abstractly. What we face, rather, are the demands that the suffering we encounter in our lives places upon us. When we are called to suffer with others (or less often to bear our own suffering), it is then that suffering becomes an issue for us. We are so selfish, so self-centered, that we simply cannot and will not begin our days by asking where we can go to relieve human misery. Even those of us in the healing professions have, at times, lost our ways and become motivated by prestige, fame, monetary reward, peer recognition, or any of a number of questionable motives rather than by the love of our hurting fellow human beings. My colleagues and I all too often complain when a clinical day is "hard" for us or we have a particularly difficult and challenging patient.

I may delude myself when I examine my own life and my personal contributions and judge that they are good. We see only our highest motives, and we feign surprise when we see abuse, violence, or civic corruption. We marvel that such abuse and transgressions could happen in our lives. We are shocked when we witness evil acts perpetrated by others, but what of our own motives? Have we never wished ill on a competitor, never spoken harshly of a colleague or corporate superior who does not embrace our plans for self-actualization, never cursed our spouse silently or openly when our needs are not met? Who in fact is good?

Admittedly, this perspective is desperately cynical. It is a view that denies all the good in the world, all the efforts of people who make true, willing sacrifices every day. It is not my wish either to be cynical or to deny the bounty of human virtue that surely exists and makes itself evident repeatedly in our lives and in our communities. I am probing, rather, what is in our hearts, at our centers, and I am trying to be honest even if it is painful. Confronting our depravity is actually an ancient question addressed by Jesus himself, and is at the center of Christian morality. What comes out of a man is what makes him "unclean": evil thoughts, sexual immorality, theft, murder, adultery, greed, malice, deceit, lewdness, envy, slander, arrogance, and folly.[18]

If what is in my heart is the delusion that I am perfect, that I am not a sinner (to use the old and now unpopular term),[19] then I will struggle endlessly with the ancient question about why I suffer. The answer is that I suffer because I am not God, because

I disobey, because my motives are impure. I am fully aware that our personal equations, our balance sheets of good versus evil, are, for most of us, tipped heavily toward the good, at least publicly. It is our private selves that hide who we are and the judgment we deserve. I believe this is one reason why we have been so consumed with our fabricated "right to privacy": in our private moments we see who we truly are, and we surely do not want others to see what we hold in our dark, private natures. We have lost the notion that what we are privately is who we are publicly. I cannot wish someone ill quietly and silently and subsequently love that person perfectly, outwardly and openly. Despite all the cancer-related suffering I see, I believe that most of the evil in the world arises from our evil motives that lead to evil deeds enacted by one person against another. Yes, there is illness. Yes, there is unexplained and seemingly illogical suffering. Much of it, though, is self-inflicted and arises from my own unwillingness to name my own sinfulness or to acknowledge that I am desperately in need of redemption.

Evil is unbearable only if there is no good. As long as the good exists, there is no ultimate problem with evil, because even though they will always exist side by side, the good is always stronger than the evil, and the good will triumph.[20] Death is tragic, in part, because of our own selfishness, because we believe it is not possible that God could minister to our lives through anyone other than the deceased. Now that they are gone, what shall we do? How can we ever be happy again? How will life be the same? We put God in a box that limits both his possibilities and ours. On the other hand, we value sacrifice and self-discipline because it mimics our patient endurance as we wait for our reward. In the words of the hymn, "Work, for the night is coming."[21]

In my defiance of God's grace, in my selfish inwardness, I deny who I am, and I deny who God is. I delude myself to imagine that I am truly good. I put God at a distance, and then I ask where he is when I suffer. Usually, he is in that figurative box in which I restrain him because I am both too ashamed and too proud to ask him to redeem my fallen, confused life. It is not surprising that I suffer, and it is no wonder I am alone, because I purposely set myself apart from God. The question "Why do bad things happen to good people?" is, of course, the question "Why do they happen to me and my loved ones?" In that question of my childish surprise lies my great denial of the reality of the suffering in our lives.

If I see ill befall another person, and I express sadness, I am really asking, "How likely is it that this bad thing (or something like it) will happen to me or someone I care about?" In the depth of my soul, I know that I am worthy of punishment for the evil that is in my heart and in my deeds, but I am not able to acknowledge this grim reality.[22] So I deny it, and I blame the suffering in the world on an absent God who is absent only because I keep him away in my denial of my fallen brokenness, in the shame of my utter depravity. Being unwilling to embrace the troubling reality of my willful separation from God, I blame him for being absent, for "sending" suffering to me. The true harshness of my suffering is not the pain itself, for that I can endure. The true agony is that I suffer alone without the knowledge that God suffers with me in my pain, that he is always present. Do I have a right to be angry about this situation?[23] My anger toward God's absence in my suffering is really an emotion substituted for my shame over my obstinate refusal to confess my sinfulness, to plead for my Father's forgiveness, and to welcome his participation in my suffering.[24]

Why Do We Suffer and Die?

So where, then, is our comfort? Have I not created a dismally and woefully pessimistic formulation of the world? After much searching and thought, I must conclude that we suffer because it is in our nature, that our suffering is part of who we are. We suffer because we are heirs of God and co-heirs with Christ, if indeed we share in his sufferings that we may also share in his glory.[25]

In our suffering, God provides us membership in his family, our promise of participation in future splendor. In that promise, he has removed the need for us to answer the great question about suffering and death. Our only remaining obligation arises out of our need to use this awareness as our sole motivation to relieve the suffering we see in others. In those acts of kindness and compassion, the great question about suffering is forever answered.

The Trappist monk Thomas Merton argued forcibly that in the incarnation, death, and resurrection of Jesus Christ, human death and suffering lost their meaning.[26] The concepts of mediation, expiation, and propitiation in the atoning death of Jesus Christ are central to the theology of the crucifixion and the resurrection, and they are essential to the recognition that suffering has no ultimate meaning of its own.[27] This is not to say that we suffer needlessly or without purpose; rather that the understanding of the purpose or end in our suffering does not have to be readily apparent or discernible by reason or logic. For those of us who believe that reasoned inquiry will bring resolution to vexing problems, the illogic of suffering confounds our intellects.[28] Merton argued, though, that faith in the abiding presence of a loving God who suffers with us is sufficient explanation for our questioning, regardless of our desire for a more satisfactory human solution.

Our Response to Suffering

An immediate consequence of a faithful recognition of God's abiding presence in suffering is our response to the suffering we see in others. If I embrace a deterministic world where events are decided by chance, it can make no possible difference whether I respond to the suffering of others. An unsatisfactory answer that has a selfish momentary appeal is the institutionalization of the caring response in civil and governmental agencies that appears to relieve me of my personal responsibility. Although this approach temporarily assuages my guilt by creating the appearance that something is being done, the response to suffering provided by institutions is often impersonal and inadequate. The only truly acceptable response to suffering is that which occurs interpersonally. Certainly, there are individuals providing care in institutional settings who respond with compassion to human suffering (as my own mother did faithfully for more than forty years as a nurse), but the institutional environment makes a personal response exceedingly difficult. Institutionalized responses to human suffering temporarily absolve our personal responsibility while making it difficult or impossible to assign blame when the caring response is inadequate. What we have overlooked in contemporary society is the personal fulfillment that comes when we respond to the needs of a sufferer: "For we pass out of death into life because we love the brethren."[29]

Should we love one another by responding to suffering because we expect some reward? The childish notion that we can somehow earn our salvation through caring for others is insufficient justification for responding to suffering. It is also a weak, fearful response that has no power at its center. No, I should not love out of a desire for reward. My response to suffering arises, instead, from a very old notion that has now lost favor in the minds of many. That is the notion of *obligation*, that we love because he first loved us.[30] The idea that we ought to respond to human suffering, the notion that we are here to do just that,[31] is an idea that runs counter to my most dearly held, fundamental, materialistic notions. Few of us espouse the belief that it is our human obligation to respond personally to suffering. It is the rare individual, indeed, who makes a personal response to suffering with little or no hope of substantial personal gain.

We in the healing professions experience significant monetary and social rewards for our efforts, and those in religious organizations labor under the promise of current or future spiritual reward. Clergy and physicians receive, for the most part, social recognition and respect for our kindnesses. What we need desperately are compassionate responses to human suffering that originate in our genuine concern for the suffering of others and are done purely for the satisfaction of having served another human being without the expectation of immediate reward. Surprisingly, this is not as difficult as it may seem.

The liberating reality is that I am free *not* to do this. I am not a puppet; I am not constrained to love anyone if I do not choose to do so. In the eternal battle between good and evil, I may choose sides. I fear that many of us no longer realize we are free to choose good because we are bombarded constantly by messages that suggest there is only evil around us. Evil does not always take the form of armies on the march or of torture in concentration camps. Rather, evil is usually more pervasive and insidious and is often manifested in everyday life by two characteristics.[32] First, it is narcissistic, seeking only to satisfy its own ends. Second, it takes human form in laziness—that is, in abject indifference to the needs of others who are suffering. This formulation of the subtleties of evil is essential to understanding our often inadequate responses to human pain.

Hatred can be defined as evil with a purpose. The evil we confront in the world is both pernicious and passive, and some of it is directed obviously and intentionally. This construction does not address the origin of all suffering, because not all suffering derives, apparently, from human evil.[33] We are certainly able to observe that some (most?) human suffering results from human evil defined as human actions following a fall from grace, the motive for which is narcissistic self-interest. This type of suffering arises from human unwillingness to seek God actively. Our unwillingness to act plays a role, I believe, even in the inner workings of "natural evil" by precluding timely preparation for predictable disaster. Among my Protestant colleagues, it is no longer fashionable to speak of the Devil. We have become too sophisticated for that sort of fantasy,[34] but when we deny the possibility of evil in human form, we lose part of our understanding of reality. Satan is our reminder that evil is powerless until it takes human form, and that it does not become hatred until it is directed specifically at another human being.

Evil that is embodied but undirected is a form of human suffering that we most commonly observe as mental illness to which M. Scott Peck devotes considerable attention. In this formulation, "natural evil" is an oxymoron, because the evil we associate with natural phenomena (such as tornadoes, earthquakes, and hurricanes) is not rooted in the phenomena themselves, but rather in our failure to provide adequate shelter before the arrival of the hurricane or after the earthquake because of our human laziness and indifference that results in human suffering. We attribute more of the suffering to the natural disaster than to our failure to create protections against its predictable consequences. This evil is our human indifference to those who live in the pall of the consequences of natural disaster, not the force of wind and rain or tumbling buildings.

Part of my apprehension of suffering arises from my unwillingness to acknowledge the existence of evil as a force in the world. If evil does not exist, explaining the effect of tangible pain such as physical suffering arising through illness becomes very difficult. Denial of evil is an extremely inefficient mechanism for dealing with its existence, however. It is far easier, nevertheless, for many of us to deny the existence of both evil and the resulting human suffering than to do the distressing and arduous work of justifying the existence of evil in a world that can seem so beautiful and desirable most of the time. The screams of individuals who are confronting the pain of sudden illness, injury, or personal loss do not arise solely from the agony of the physical or emotional suffering, but equally from our reluctant acquiescence to the fact that pain and suffering are realities of the creation. It is easier for me to deny the Fall or to dismiss it merely as a literary curiosity than to plumb the profound implications of my willful separation from a compassionate creator. Another terrible consequence of suffering is the loneliness that it imparts or forces upon us. This loneliness demands that we take an account of who we are and what we have been when illness, pain, and suffering arrive. If this searching takes place for the first time after decades of unexamined living, physical suffering is further compounded by the emotional torment of coming face-to-face with the regrets of one's life and an accompanying feeling of worrisome guilt.

The solutions to human suffering are available in the creation, but evil has kept us from diligently seeking the answers to these problems. The serendipity of scientific discovery is one possible demonstration of the willingness of God to provide relief of our suffering if we will allow ourselves to be agents of his will.[35] I realize with St. Paul that I do what I do not want to do,[36] and I find myself suffering as a result. Our failures to relieve suffering in others arise more often from the immobility that is caused by our fears than from the evil that is in us. Therefore, our response to suffering must be compassionate love, because perfect love drives out fear.[37]

---

[1] Kübler-Ross, E. *Death: The Final Stage of Growth*. New York: Scribner Simon & Schuster, 2009.

[2] Kelly RJ, Smith TJ. Delivering maximum clinical benefit at an affordable price: engaging stakeholders in cancer care. *Lancet Oncology* 2014;15:e112-118.

[3] Sadly, health is not assured for a great majority of the world's population who are born into sickness and suffering and are never really well.

[4] Selby-Bigge LA (ed.). *Enquiries Concerning the Human Understanding and Concerning the Principles of Morals by David Hume*. New York: Oxford University Press, 1970.

[5] Abernethy AP, Kamal AH. "Palliative and end-of-life care" in Loprinzi CL (editor). ASCO-SEP: Medical oncology self-evaluation program, Third Edition. American Society of Clinical Oncology, Inc. Alexandria, VA, 2013, 499-523

[6] Matthew 10:39.

[7] 2 Corinthians 11:3.

[8] Hebrews 11:1.

9. Hebrews 3.
10. Physicists have identified the Weak Anthropic Principle (Hawking S. *A Brief History of Time*. Bantam Doubleday Dell, New York, 1998) that says, in effect, that the universe was designed with man as its chief end. Even minor changes in the laws of the physical universe would make it impossible for the appearance or the continuation of humanity. See also Tippler FJ. *The Physics of Immortality*. New York: Anchor Books, 1995.
11. Isaac Newton, *Principia Mathematica*, 2nd edition, 1713.
12. Exodus 3:14.
13. E.g. the Spanish Inquisition.
14. Psalm 1:6, Proverbs 11:10, Proverbs 28:28, Isaiah 57:1.
15. Kushner H. *Why Do Bad Things Happen to Good People?* New York: Schocken Books, 1989.
16. Ibid.
17. Marty M. *Martin Luther*. New York: Viking Penguin, 2004, 77.
18. Mark 7:18–23.
19. Menninger K. *Whatever Became of Sin?* New York: Hawthorne, 1973.
20. Frankl, Viktor. *Man's Search for Meaning*. New York: Washington Square Press, 1998.
21. "Work, for the night is coming" Work, for the night is coming Under the sunset skies; While their bright tints are glowing, Work, for daylight flies;" By Annie Louise Coghill, 1854. http://www.hymnary.org/text/work_for_the_night_is_coming (Accessed September 13, 2014)
22. 2 Samuel 12:1–12.
23. Jonah 4:4.
24. Sören Kierkegaard explained this in *The Sickness Unto Death*. Princeton, NJ: Princeton University Press, 1941. The sickness for him was despair. The remedy for despair is to embrace, through faith, that we are created and loved by God who participates in our suffering.
25. "The Spirit himself testifies with our spirit that we are God's children. Now if we are children, then we are heirs—heirs of God and co-heirs with Christ, if indeed we share in his sufferings in order that we may also share in his glory. I consider that our present sufferings are not worth comparing with the glory that will be revealed in us." Romans 8:16–18.
26. Merton was born January 31, 1915, in Prades, France. His early education was in England and France, and he earned degrees at Columbia University in 1938 and 1939. After teaching English at Columbia (1938–39) and at St. Bonaventure University (1939–41),

he entered the Trappist Abbey of Gethsemani near Louisville, Kentucky, where he was ordained as a priest in 1949. Merton's first published works were collections of poems, but international fame came to him after the publication of his autobiographical *Seven Storey Mountain* (New York: Harcourt Brace & Co., 1948 and 1998). He was electrocuted by a faulty wire during an international monastic convention in Bangkok, Thailand, in December 1968.

[27] Merton T. *No Man Is an Island.* New York: Harcourt, Brace Jovanovich, 1983, 78.

"Suffering is consecrated to God by faith—not by faith in suffering but by faith in God. Suffering has no power and no value of its own. It is valuable only as a test of faith."

"The mercy of God is given to those who seek Him in suffering, and by His grace we can overcome evil with good. Suffering, then, becomes good by accident, by the good that it enables us to receive more abundantly from the mercy of God… Thus, what we consecrate to God in suffering is not our suffering but our selves."

[28] The word of the cross is foolishness to them that perish, but to them that are saved it is the power of God (I Corinthians 1:18).
[29] 1 John 3:14. Frankl, Viktor. Ibid.
[30] 1 John 4:19.
[31] John 13:34.
[32] Peck, MS. *People of the Lie: The Hope for Healing Human Evil.* New York: Simon and Schuster, 1998.
[33] St. Augustine argued that God could not have created evil, he being, himself, totally good. Evil, therefore, was seen to derive from humanity's fall, including the evil that is inherent in the creation, such as earthquakes, tornadoes, volcanoes, etc. This is a metaphysical argument beyond the scope of the present discussion of the human response to human suffering, independent of its origins.
[34] Pegels E. *The Origin of Satan: How Christians Demonized Jews, Pagans, and Heretics.* New York: Vintage Press, 1996.
[35] Matthew 7:7.
[36] Romans 7:19.
[37] There is no fear in love. But perfect love drives out fear, because fear has to do with punishment. The one who fears is not made perfect in love. (1 John 4:18)

11

We Happy Few: Sharing Grief with Friends

> To believe is nothing other than to think with assent ... believers are also thinkers: in believing, they think and in thinking, they believe. If faith does not think, it is nothing. If there is no assent, there is no faith, for without assent one does not really believe.[1]
> —St. Augustine

Our friendship with Rolf and his children did not end with Hilda's untimely death. Rolf and his daughter Katharina visited us for the Fourth of July seven months after Hilda died. It was a painful visit that we wished would have been more joyous. Their visit brought melancholy where, just a year earlier, we had all hoped for merriment. We shared stories from Rolf and Hilda's first visit. We showed Katharina the terra cotta pot Hilda had brought us from Mexico. We filled it with flowers that we called "Hilda's geraniums." On July 4 we all rode bicycles in the neighborhood parade, and there was something delightfully ironic about a German friend and his daughter wearing red, white, and blue and pedaling bicycles accompanied by recorded John Philip Sousa marches playing from loudspeakers. After the bicycle parade we ate watermelon and then went home for a proper and festive Fourth of July picnic.

On Sunday we invited Rolf to our church. Our Sunday school class was studying the Gospel of John, and Rolf brought his German Bible with him. As the pages lay open to "Johannes," Rolf admitted that he was struggling to believe the good news of the gospel, and his pain was evident. I agonized with him both silently and openly, rolling around in my mind my own doubts and frustrations about my mother's death. My only comfort was that Rolf knew I could ache with him and his loss of Hilda in my torment over the loss of my mother.

Before Hilda died, Rolf had called me to ask one last time if I had any additional treatments to offer her. In the most reassuring way that I knew, I told him that we had very few effective therapies to control metastatic breast cancer at the time and none to cure it. Shortly afterward, Rolf called my home in Houston late on a Friday evening. He sometimes had trouble finding me in my office so he learned to call after midnight in Germany, which usually found me at home for dinner. This time, I was out of town on a business trip, and Sally spoke to him for quite a while. When she told me about her conversation with Rolf, she was visibly excited. She had been so moved by Rolf's remarks that she took notes to refresh her memory.

When Hilda and Rolf visited us in those few months before her death, we, of course, had many meals together. It is customary in our home to say grace before meals, and I did not alter our practice when the Mullers visited. Rolf told Sally that these prayers had made a great impression on him, as did our prayers at church.

These were not prayers for Hilda specifically, and we did not try to heal her through intercessory prayer or the laying on of hands. We prayed only the simple prayers one prays before a meal and the prayers of church worship. As a result of these simple acts, Rolf said he wrote a protocol (like a document describing the experimental investigation of a new drug) to offer prayer each hour to bring God's power to Hilda. He said that Hilda's mother used to pray, and that when his mother-in-law died four months before Hilda, he believed that prayer became his duty. He said he came to believe through these prayers that Hilda's time after her earthly life was no different from her life on earth. He said that Hilda was very happy during the last few weeks of her life, and that her illness was a "happy adventure."

During his July visit to our home, he brought with him a picture of Hilda and a friend walking through the autumn foliage in the Sauerland woods near the clinic at Mischwald. The sky is gray and the woods are dark, but Hilda's coat is bright red, and she is carrying a red umbrella. They both speak an unstated silent peace that she felt and reported to Rolf and others. On the back of the picture, Rolf wrote the following: "Hilda's (in red) last walk near the Veramed clinic, Meschede, in November. It seems she is already on her way into a better area. Taken by Rolf and according to Hilda, given to good friends in Houston."

I have no idea how this peace transcended, but I do not doubt at all that it happened. When Rolf tried to explain it to Sally, he referred to Heather's brief essay about her father being a hero. To my surprise, he said I was not a hero because I do cancer research; rather, I was a hero to him because I go to church. My simple witness of prayers at the dinner table and an invitation to the husband of a patient to attend church with me had made all the difference in the way he accepted her death. I believe we often look for far more complex answers when simple ones will suffice. Let us pray for a bit of simplicity.

Epilogue

I stayed in contact with Rolf through the years, mostly with Christmas letters. Seven years after Hilda died, Sally and I had an opportunity to return to Europe with Heather and Chris. We advised Rolf of our plans to visit the continent, and he insisted that we come to Aurich. He said he had, in his words, "a lady friend" whom he wanted us to meet. Her name was Maria.

We flew from Philadelphia to Amsterdam and spent the weekend as tourists. We rented a Volvo station wagon and made the five-hour drive through the Dutch countryside along the coast of the North Sea into Friesland. Sally and I hardly knew what to expect, returning so many years after our first visit, and this time with our children, but any fears we had were ill-founded. Rolf had now married Maria, and she was quite gracious even when we spoke repeatedly of Hilda, perhaps because she was a widow, too, and had known the painful loss of her lifetime companion.

We had a lovely visit touring Aurich and the surrounding countryside, mostly with Rolf, but occasionally with Maria as well. We had dinner with friends of theirs in Aurich and in Leer, the nearby port town. We even visited Hilda's grave in a quiet rural cemetery. Rolf was most proud to show us the high school that he called the "gymnasium" where he taught business classes. We spent a day on Rolf's sailboat that we had visited with Hilda when she was ill, but this time we made a day trip to the island of Baltrum in the North Sea, and Heather and Chris took turns at the helm of the sturdy sailing craft. During our brief voyage, we passed sea lions sunning themselves on the beach of a small island, and it all seemed very peaceful. On Baltrum, the hearty Rolf and our brave Chris weathered the icy water of the North Sea for a brief swim. It was all great fun, and shared with such casualness and comfort that we might have been mistaken for lifelong friends.

Rolf was happy to escort us on a driving tour of central Germany, and we stopped to visit Katharina at the University of Münster, where she was a student. We then visited the thirteenth-century castle called Berg Els in the Mosel River valley. During our tour of the massive edifice, I found myself repeatedly humming the hymn tune "A Mighty Fortress Is Our God" and thinking persistently of Martin Luther. We toured small, romantic towns such as Bernkastel and Cochem along the river that is lined with rich vineyards rising steeply above the nearly vertical banks of the valley. It is from these vineyards that the wines labeled "Mosel-Saar-Ruer" originate. We even saw the "Schwartz Katz" painted on a wall in the town famous for its Black Cat wines. At Burg we met Rolf's dear friend who is the proprietor of the Hotel Zur Post, where we enjoyed a five-star meal followed by wine tasting in the cellar of the grand old establishment.

On one level, our friendship with Rolf made no sense. I had been the doctor far away in America to whom he had brought Hilda with so much hope; I had disappointed him, and now we had Hilda no more. Once during our visit when I mentioned some of the research in breast cancer prevention that I was doing, hoping to be optimistic and encouraging, Rolf said immediately, "Yes, but it is too late for Hilda, and it will not help your mother." I could sense the pain in his voice, yet he was neither bitter nor caustic. He merely told me how lonely it was to live without Hilda after being with her for so many years. I understood perfectly, because Rolf's pain and emptiness was the same pain that I had experienced after losing my mother. That, in fact, was what we shared, what linked us across the ocean, different languages, and historically warring cultures: that common experience of having shared the painful journey that is the loss of a loved one and having come out on the other side feeling a kinship like that known by warriors who have survived the battlefield.

October 25 is the feast of St. Crispin. On that day in 1415, King Henry V of England with 2,000 cavalry and 13,000 of his countrymen defeated 60,000 Frenchmen at the Battle of Agincourt. Before the battle, King Henry rallied his troops by arguing convincingly that though they were greatly outnumbered, they were a privileged few who would be the envy of their countrymen for having prevailed in battle:

> This story shall the good man teach his son; And Crispin Crispian shall ne'er go by, From this day to the ending of the world, But we in it shall be remembered— We few, we happy few, we band of brothers; For he today that sheds his blood with me Shall be my brother; be he ne'er so vile, This day shall gentle his condition; And gentlemen in England, now a-bed, Shall think themselves accurs'd they were not here; And hold their manhoods cheap whiles any speaks That fought with us upon Saint Crispin's day. [2]

The French lost 7,000 men in the battle; the English, 500.

Rolf and I had shed figurative blood together, and now we were bothers bound in a grim fraternity where no one willingly seeks membership, but where each knows that having passed the initiation rite of painful loss, the camaraderie is deep and profound, and the friendship is lifelong. We all embraced warmly as we departed, hoping there would be another visit soon.

On Faith

Christian Scripture tells us that faith is being sure of what we hope for and certain of what we do not see.[3] Conversely, one of the defining intellectual and spiritual realities of the nineteenth and twentieth centuries was scientific skepticism, and Rolf was well versed in this doubt.[4] Ironically, we believe only what we can know through an accepted system of evidence and proofs, yet we seldom question the fundamental wisdom of the system or the rules whereby we gather our understanding. If we stray outside the system, accepting what we know without questioning, taking beliefs on faith, being subjective and not objective, our deductive colleagues in rigorous scientific circles will label us naive and foolish (or even dangerous).

Recent cultural and societal experience bolsters skepticism toward those who espouse faith in things not seen. Faith is tainted by those who use it for monetary gain or political advantage, or by those caught in religious hypocrisy. Yet faith, of all the virtues, is most central to a meaningful and lastingly successful confrontation with death. Where faith dies, all hope is lost; where hope is lost, men and women create and accept belief systems that cannot ultimately succeed and that require increasingly complex rationalizations to maintain and defend them. Where faith dies, hope dies, and along with it, God dies as a possibility in the mind of the skeptic. There follows a desperation and yearning that propels us along a journey on which we search for imperfect solutions that cannot redeem our longing for unity and completeness.

Fear of death is a logical consequence of a belief system in which human intellect must provide answers that can be rightly provided only through the revelation that follows, that comes as a consequence of, belief. Logic is ultimately defeated in any attempt to defend or rationally refute the existence of God. Faith is faith only when it alone will suffice. If appeals to logic yield answers to a particular problem, we are not dealing in matters of faith. Faith begins at the limits of human understanding and takes us to an assurance in things we can imagine in part but cannot fully comprehend.

We are incapacitated by fear and misunderstanding about death. Our fear is the bondage that prevents us from loving ourselves and loving each other. It is only in confronting and overcoming our fear of death that we become free to love. Only in that love can we truly serve, and only in that service do we obtain the fulfillment we so desperately seek. When we look through the hideous yet transparent monster that is death, our human eyes see nothingness on the other side. This nothingness is the source of our most profound terror, a terror that sends us running, for most of our lives, in directions that avoid confrontation with the enemy, death. As we run, we blindly bypass opportunities to love others, and in doing so, to fulfill ourselves. We substitute opportunities to love others who are suffering with puny, inadequate attempts to avoid death that do not satisfy our yearning to love and to be loved.

Doctor, What if it Were Your Mother?

The avoidance of our own mortality, and, therein, the mortality and suffering of those around us is a moral tragedy of our generation. I believe that no solution designed to serve the needs of others can be adequate without first addressing our calamitous failure to confront death and suffering or to provide an adequate response to their pain. Curiously, it is my experience that if we identify practical means whereby we can respond adequately to the suffering we see, we are liberated to a higher plane of extraordinary possibilities. Death becomes not the adversary to be combated but the ultimate portal through which we are ushered into the holy presence of God. This meeting is neither to be feared nor embraced hurriedly or unadvisedly, but rather to be welcomed without fear at the duly appointed time.

During my many trips to Europe I often contemplated the arduous flight of the *Spirit of St. Louis* from the quiet security of my business-class seat, comfortable and safe as I reclined more than thirty thousand feet above the ocean. Charles Lindbergh planned his Atlantic crossing meticulously. He drew his projected course on the latest available navigational charts. He estimated his time en route using his previously calculated true airspeed plus estimated wind velocity and direction. He updated his estimates by noting the time of passage of each checkpoint and recalculated his ground speed and estimated time remaining to his destination. His methods are still used today by pilots who fly with far more sophisticated navigational equipment. Despite Lindbergh's logic and intellect, despite his careful planning and calculations and recalculations during the flight, he began to have doubts about finding land just before dawn near the end of his strenuous crossing. He wrote that as the hours grew longer, he questioned whether Europe was there at all! He wrestled with himself in his fatigue and convinced himself that "It [Europe] must be there. The charts show it. They didn't lie about Nova Scotia. They told the truth about Newfoundland. I've measured them accurately. Europe must be there too. I know people who have been to Europe."[5]

Indeed, he knew such people. In his fatigue and anxious longing to sight land, Lindbergh forgot that he knew with certainty that Europe was where it was. Of course, that was his very reason for being in this small plane for more than twenty hours over the Atlantic. In his fatigue and desperate longing for the ordeal to be concluded, he told himself he knew Europe was there because of the reports of other people. He didn't need their testimony, but he desperately tried to persuade himself through logic to accept something he had already accepted through faith: that Europe lay twenty-three hours east of St. John's, Newfoundland, for the *Spirit of St. Louis* and for him. No testimony could prove that for him, no logic could convince him of that fact, because no plane had ever done it before. It was by faith that he prevailed. Yet the question of faith troubled Lindbergh for years after the historic flight:

> The problems continued to throb in my mind through years beyond childhood. Is there a God? Is there an existence after life? Is there something within one's body that doesn't age with years? There were times when I considered taking up the study of biology and medicine so I could explore the mysteries of life and death. But these sciences belonged to well-grounded, brilliant minds; their study was intricate, and my school marks were poor in subjects they demanded as a background ... Being a physician, great-grandfather Edwin must have

lived in close contact with both life and death. There didn't seem to be any conflict in his mind between science and God. His studies of biology didn't convince him that all existence ends with the flesh. He had faith in some quality that is independent of the body.[6]

Flying on instruments without reference to identifiable landmarks is a test of faith. Flying in the clouds ("in the soup" in aviation vernacular) or above a low-lying, featureless cloud deck requires both concentration and faith. When there are no references, when the outside visible horizon is replaced by a gyroscopically driven artificial horizon on the instrument panel, and when there are no visible checkpoints by which to measure progress, instrument flying truly becomes a test of faith.

For the novice instrument pilot, the lack of visual references can lead to spatial disorientation through reliance on his own senses rather than on the instruments. Acceleration and deceleration lead to erroneous sensual indications of turning, and a stable, nonaccelerating turn gives no perceptible sensations to the unwary pilot. Relying on the logic of the senses will lead ultimately to disaster for any pilot who attempts to maintain directional and positional control through this mechanism. The instrument pilot must make a conscious effort to ignore physical sensations during flight without outside visual references.

Similarly, a life without faith leads to a loss of directional control and the inevitable "graveyard spiral." Faith emboldens us in a manner like the confidence possessed by the instrument pilot who puts faith in the instruments and not in his senses. With faith, the pilot will attempt things confidently that the non-instrument pilot would be terrified to contemplate, let alone attempt.

How does one acquire faith that empowers? First, by acknowledging that there are forces in control of the universe (defined as God for many) that impart a logic and order that defy complete human understanding. The compassion and love of God directs these forces for our ultimate good even through the pain of death. Second, we admit with the saints that "we are aliens and strangers on earth"[7] who long for a better country—a heavenly one.[8] The instrument pilot cannot see his destination when he begins. In fact, he often cannot see the next checkpoint or even the current one. He knows only that his instruments say that he has arrived at his checkpoint, and they point him to the next one. Only faith in the instruments, denial of the senses, and belief in his ultimate plan will allow the instrument pilot to arrive at his destination.

I have made flights during which I lost sight of the ground within thirty seconds of takeoff and did not regain visual contact with the ground until thirty seconds before touchdown. The hours in between have been punctuated by encounters with icing, thunderstorms, lost communications, and much anxiety. Only faith in the system, my flight plan, the airplane, and its instruments have sustained me as an instrument pilot.

So it is with death. Many of the sensory cues that come to us about death are false. Despite the popular depictions of death as grotesque and horrible, in my clinical experience, an individual's terror of death is greater with greater distance from it. It is important to make a distinction here between suffering and death. Suffering is grotesque and horrible; pain is noxious and is to be avoided. Although much of the work of the physician who deals with dying patients is properly spent in the relief of physical suffering, we consider here, rather, the imagined anxieties that people experience *in anticipation* of death. The most intense anxieties about dying I have seen are found in patients who are very far from dying and are unlikely to die: the young woman with a fractured leg sustained in an automobile accident or the heart attack victim whose vital signs are stable forty-eight hours after the event. Usually, their anxiety comes from their seriously and personally contemplating death for the first time in their lives.

I have seen intense anxiety in the family members of the recently deceased and in those who are about to die. Yet, just as faith in flight instruments leads to directed, purposeful flight in the absence of visual cues, so, too, does faith in God lead to confidence in the face of death. The faith of the ancients "conquered kingdoms, administered justice, and gained what was promised; [it] shut the mouths of lions, quenched the fury of the flames, and escaped the edge of the sword; [their] weakness was turned to strength; and [they] became powerful in battle."[9] Faith tells us that

> "... neither death nor life, neither angels or demons, neither the present or the future, nor any powers, neither height nor depth, nor anything else in all creation, will be able to separate us from the love of God that is in Christ Jesus our Lord."[10]

Shortly before his death, my father asked his brother Donald to read those words at his memorial service, which he did tearfully and with great faith.

Death that is approached with this certainty, with this assurance, with this faith, becomes a conquered foe. Once this foe is conquered, once we are confident of the loving presence of the redeeming God, no anxiety or fear can prevent us from setting out on our most challenging tasks. This is not to say that we will never experience tragedy, never crash and burn our fragile crafts. Faith does not insulate us from calamity, and it is a childish and immature faith that believes this to be true. But faith in God, like faith in the instruments of the pilot, makes the likelihood of encountering tragedy alone and helpless almost impossible. Tragedy will come, as do cloudy days with poor visibility and low ceilings. But by faith, God most assuredly sees us through tragedy to a bright and glorious victory.

---

[1] St. Augustine quoted in *Fides et Ratio*, Encyclical Letter of the Supreme Pontiff John Paul II to the Bishops of the Catholic Church on the Relationship between Faith and Reason, page 68. http://www.vatican.va/holy_father/john_paul_ii/encyclicals/documents/hf_jp-ii_enc_15101998_fides-et-ratio_en.html (Accessed September 13, 2014)

[2] Shakespeare, William. *Henry V*, Act IV, Scene III. Crispin and Crispinian were early Christian martyrs and the patron saints of shoemakers

[3] Hebrews 11:1,2

[4] Hecht, Jennifer Michael. *Doubt—a History*. New York: Harper Collins, 2004.

[5] Lindbergh, Charles A. *The Spirit of St. Louis*, New York: Charles Scribner's & Sons, 1953, 459.

[6] Ibid., pp. 319-321

[7] Hebrews 11:13

[8] Hebrews 11:16

[9] Hebrews 11:33, 34

[10] Romans 8:38, 39

12

Contemplating Suffering and Doubt from a Distance

> These days the biggest temple and mosque and gurudwara
> is the place where man works for the good of mankind.
> —Jawaharial Nehru (sign in the New Delhi Airport Domestic Terminal)

Western government, science, scholarship, and theater all had their origins in Athens. From Democritus in the fifth century BC we received the Atomist theory that anticipated John Locke's distinction between primary and secondary qualities of matter. We learned oration from Desmosthenes; medicine from Hippocrates and Diocles; philosophy from Plato, Aristotle, Epicurus and countless others; tragic theater from Aeschylus, Sophocles, and Euripides; architecture and sculpture from Ictinus and Phidias, designer and sculptor of the Parthenon; statesmanship from Pericles; and the science of history from Thucydides.

Athens was at the center of Western culture from its beginning. Settlements on the southern slopes of the Acropolis date from 3000

BC, and the Acropolis became a fortified royal citadel covering an area of 35,000 square meters as early as 1400 BC. The oligarchic state emerged in the eighth century BC, and by the middle of the fifth century BC, the Greeks had defeated the Persians and established themselves as a dominant military power. After the defeat of the Persians, the Athenians began to erect most of the structures of the current Acropolis on the rubble left behind by the defeated Persians. The Parthenon was completed between 437 and 438 BC and stands today as an enduring monument to a civilization and a culture that established the institutions we have inherited, often without thought or reflection or gratitude for the Greek legacy.[1]

The most favorable way to explore a new city is on foot. With guidebook in hand, it is a pleasure to explore the most intimate scenes of strange locales without a guide or a predetermined plan. Sally and I have done this in Amsterdam, Nice, Paris, Monaco, Hamburg, Berlin, Rhodes, Rome, and London. In this way, it is possible to find shops and restaurants, statues and cathedrals, parks and fountains that might otherwise be impossible to discover. On a walking tour, one can linger over the delightful and the fascinating.

Athens holds much to see on a casual afternoon stroll. The market, or *plaka,* is a group of shops and restaurants packed in a jostle of competing togetherness reminiscent of the ancient markets. It encircles the base of the Acropolis towering majestically above the noise and activity of the eager shoppers. There are leather goods and pottery, china and brass, lace and linen, and innumerable religious icons of the Greek Orthodox faith. Much of this remains unchanged after centuries, guarded in silent splendor by the temples of the Acropolis, decayed little by the passage of time.

The path from the *plaka* to the summit of the Acropolis tracks along a gradually rising walkway that winds lazily through juniper and cedar bushes. On the southern slope of the fabled hill are two mammoth amphitheaters whose stone stages and seats are but slightly worn by two and a half millennia of weather, barbarian invaders, theatergoers, and tourists. If one is silent while sitting on the stone seats, it seems possible to hear faint echoes of a Thucidean tragedy entertaining the learned patrons of centuries ago. In great cathedrals and country churches, in wooded chapels and suburban shrines, I have sensed the presence of God. In this place, I was not touched by a feeling of God's presence, but rather by the whispered murmurings of great minds now long silent. This was not a holy place, yet it was filled with echoes of great cognitive confrontations, of profound struggles of men espousing great ideals and morals and new methods of government. It was a cathedral of reasoning.

Sally and I walked along the path at the southern boundary of the Acropolis toward the entrance of the Parthenon. Our meanderings took us past the Odeion of Herodes Atticus, a huge open-air theater in the Roman style. The three dozen rows of marble seats held an audience of 5,000 that dwarfed the nearby Greek theater of Dionysos. This smaller amphitheater is 400 years older than the Odeion and is named for the seat in the center of the first row reserved for the priest of Dionysos Eleuthereus. It was in this theater that Greek tragedy had its birth, and Aeschylus, Sophocles and Euripides all appeared in person.

We made our way up the path and peered into the Parthenon. As I contemplated the countless generations who had looked on what I was now seeing, I felt as though I were receiving a cultural and intellectual legacy, a gift of thought and beauty that was passed quietly and soberly along through centuries of conflict, strife, tradition, and hope. As fascinating as it was, though, this was a temple of idols. Some of the idols still stood, and some had great and enduring physical beauty, but no souls were there to worship them.

Sally and I knew that the apostle Paul had come to Athens on his third missionary journey. He waited in Athens for Silas and Timothy to join him so that the three of them could continue their journey together. Paul had enjoyed some success with his preaching in Thessalonica and was able to convince "a large number of God-fearing Greeks and not a few prominent women of the truth of the Gospel."[2] According to the text, "While Paul was waiting for them in Athens, he was greatly distressed to see that the city was full of idols. So he reasoned in the synagogue with the Jews and the God-fearing Greeks, as well as in the marketplace day by day with those who happened to be there."[3] We also knew from the text that he had taught in the Areopagus, the court of the city. Paul's teaching of the life of Christ puzzled the Greeks, and they asked him, "May we know what this new teaching is that you are presenting? You are bringing some strange ideas to our ears, and we want to know what they mean." The Athenians and the foreigners who lived there spent their time doing nothing but talking about and listening to the latest ideas. So in this forum of ideas, Paul stood up in the meeting of the Areopagus and said, "Men of Athens! I see that in every way you are very religious. For as I walked around and looked carefully at your objects of worship, I even found an altar with this inscription: *To an unknown god.*

Now what you worship as something unknown I am going to proclaim to you."

Faith was meeting reason and speaking the logic it both knew and understood.

Paul explained that the God who made the world and everything in it is the Lord of heaven and earth, and that he does not live in temples built by human hands. He is the giver of all life and breath and everything else we humans have, and he sets before us the ways of life and death. God did this so that men would seek him and even reach out for him and find him, though he is not far from each one of us. To show the learned Greeks that he was knowledgeable about history and literature, Paul quoted a saying attributed to either Minos or Epimenedes of Crete: "For in him we live and move and have our being."[4] He also quoted the poet Aratus of Cilicia, who said, "We are his offspring." Having laid the foundation for the argument, Paul completed the syllogism: "Therefore since we are God's offspring, we should not think that the divine being is like gold or silver or stone—an image made by man's design and skill. In the past God overlooked such ignorance, but now he commands all people everywhere to repent. For he has set a day when he will judge the world with justice by the man he has appointed. He has given proof of this to all men by raising him from the dead."[5]

We had come all the way to Athens, and Sally and I wanted to see the place where Paul had made his famous speech to the ancient Athenians. Areopagus means "Hill of Ares or Mars," and it was the seat of the supreme court of ancient Athens. According to mythical tradition Ares was called to account by the gods for the murder of Halirrhotios, and here Orestes stood trial for the murder of his mother, Klytaimnestra. In the fifth century BC, the

Areopagus was reduced to a constitutional court and a court of morals. I wanted to see this place where the apostle wrestled with the greatest intellectuals of his age for the purpose of telling them the Good News. It was, of course, the most radical (and to some, the most outlandish) idea they had ever heard.

As we searched for this famous place, it occurred to me how my modern intellectual friends in academia were just like the Athenians, and I thought that seeing the Areopagus would give me some coveted insight I did not yet possess, some ammunition for the verbal battles yet to be fought with the doubting intellectuals and scientists at home.

Our guidebook was not clear about where the Areopagus actually was, placing it somewhere "northwest of the Acropolis." On the map this was a very large area, almost as large as the Acropolis itself. As we wandered off in the general direction of northwest, we had very little idea of where we were going and a very difficult time finding signs or other markings. We wandered through streets and narrow driveways, stopping occasionally to ask shopkeepers if they knew the location of the fabled Areopagus. Most of them had never heard of it, and not one knew where it was. Local natives were puzzled. Other tourists had no idea.

As we wandered more and more to the southwest now, we approached the Hill of the Muses, where we got a spectacular and famous view of the Acropolis atop the hill that is almost 500 feet above sea level. Near there, we wandered past a wedding party that was just leaving a small chapel. When the bride saw our camera, she smiled and agreed to have her picture taken. I told her the picture would be going all the way back to Texas, and she smiled even more broadly and beamed, "I'm Italian!" We thanked her and smiled back, embracing her joy for a moment before we continued to search, winding our way back to the northwest side of the Acropolis.

Suddenly, a stiff wind arose and blew debris into my eyes, lodging under my contact lenses and causing me to squint severely and temporarily lose my vision. After much blinking and tearing, I slowly opened my eyes without pain so that I could continue our search. As we walked, I recalled how St. Paul himself had been blinded briefly by God for the purpose of gaining insight into God's calling for him.[6] As I stumbled about in my own "blindness," we came upon a rock very near where we had begun our search for the Areopagus. On it was a plaque written in Greek that marked the place of the famous court. We had searched the hill of the Acropolis when what we were looking for had literally been in front of us the entire time. We had been searching for a plaque written in English while standing in the heart of Greek culture and society. I realized how foolish we must be at times, searching vainly for resolution to our troubling questions while overlooking the answers placed before us.

If we will simply open our eyes, we will see.

Yet another perspective

Several years later, I had another chance to look back toward American culture and values from the unique vantage and perspectives that come from being on the other side of the world. Because we had such a wonderful experience at the biennial meeting of the UICC in Hamburg, Germany years earlier, when Sally and I learned that the UICC would meet in New Delhi, India, we were eager to make the trip to see the exotic subcontinent firsthand. I was to present a paper about screening young women at risk for breast cancer with mammography. Preparations included a series of immunizations and the requirement to take malaria prophylaxis before and after the trip. I thought this was a bit curious given that we were to visit only major cities, but we complied. The conference organizers made a number of post-meeting trips available, and we agreed that if we had come all this distance, we were going to take in as many sights as possible.

What we do in North America with machinery, India does with manual labor. We observed the excavation of a foundation for a house hewn in solid rock with picks and shovels by elderly women who were carrying out the loose rock in baskets and metal pans balanced on their heads. No front-end loader or backhoe was in evidence anywhere. Heavily laden donkeys transported bricks and sand through the old city of Udaipur to a construction site. In some places, including the city streets in Jaipur and Udaipur, "holy cows" assembled in herds in city plazas, and everywhere the citizens were as unimpressed by the presence of the cows as the cows were by the pedestrians and the vehicular traffic that pressed their way through the narrow streets. The cows wandered lazily over the streets, eating scraps from piles of garbage and fallen marigold leis or ritual corn left at the Buddhist temples by believers who profess that it is sacred to feed the animals.

Travel on the streets and roads in this environment is unsettling to most Westerners. The British custom of driving on the left side of the road initiates the disorientation, and the crowding completes it. An unwritten law of the road dictates that the slower jitneys yield to the larger, faster vehicles. Pedestrians and cyclists move near the berm of the road, apparently oblivious to the imminent danger moving at forty kilometers an hour just a few feet away. Motorized rickshaws beep a cricket cough to warn pedestrians of the traffic overtaking them from behind. Most harrowing is the passage of oncoming trucks and buses whose sheer bulk makes safe side-by-side passage a challenge on such narrow causeways. There were no lines painted on the highways, which were both rough and uneven. There was frequent road construction, but there were no construction signs, no highly visible barriers, no orange barrels, no blinking lights, not even old-style flame pots. Survival on the road in India came through keen alertness and extraordinary coordination of large vehicles dancing a near catastrophic weave at high speed in desperate proximity to each other.

A bus overtaking slower traffic swings out into the oncoming lane of traffic, all the while wailing the mandatory beep-beep-beep that warns the slower traffic to give way to the left. Inevitably, the overtaking bus meets oncoming traffic, usually a TATA-brand Indian truck. Just as it appeared that this mechanized test of the drivers' nerve and resolve would result in a massive collision, both the slower traffic on the left and the overtaking traffic in the passing lane on the right found accommodating spaces, averting tragedy with barely inches to spare. This mechano-waltz was repeated at slower speed in the crowded city streets, where pedestrian traffic scooted across the boulevards in front of oncoming traffic, seemingly unaware of the onrushing danger and yet aware each moment of the danger of being struck. The cars, buses, and trucks lurched and weaved, beeping madly at pedestrians who persisted in their courses and never appeared to flinch as danger passed so nearby.

The Taj Mahal may be the most famous building in the world, and it was the one sight in India we wanted to see most. It is in

Agra, Uttar Pradesh, a city 220 kilometers (about 137 miles) from Delhi, but getting to Agra was one of the most challenging trips we have ever made. The organizers told us we had two options. We could ride the train, but that meant we were on our own when we arrived in Agra, and that did not seem wise. The other choice was to ride a bus with a guide. It sounded like the better plan. Then we got the details. The bus would leave Delhi at 5:00 a.m. We would stop along the way for breakfast, proceed to Agra, have a guided tour of the Taj Mahal, and then return to Delhi on the bus. We were told it would be a "nice day trip," and we eagerly joined twenty others for the adventure. We were astonished when the bus trip took over five hours one-way to complete.

Imagine every conceivable conveyance: bicycles, wooden carts, tractors pulling wagons, "steam rollers," scooters, motorcycles, motorized rickshaws, bicycle rickshaws, donkeys, camel carts, yoked oxen, horse carts, TATA trucks. Now, imagine every kind of person walking along a road: children, women bearing bundles on their heads, old men shuffling slowly. Add to the scene a veritable bestiary of nonhuman forms: camels, cows, goats, pigs, dogs, cats, monkeys, elephants. Just for amusement, add snake charmers with cobras in baskets, a handler of a boa constrictor, and men with bears and monkeys on leashes performing at the masters' commands, always ready to pose for the lucrative photo with the reluctant and astonished tourist. We observed all this both before and during our five-hour bus ride to Agra.

Agra is a crowded city of more than 1.5 million people with no directional traffic or street signs. The choked streets are lined by small, dirty roadside vendors selling every manner of produce and goods. At the Agra Fort, a 500-year-old monument to the victorious Mogul emperors from the Muslim empires to the west, there were amputees begging for alms and a boy with massive lymphedema of his feet. The condition, probably caused by parasitic worms obstructing the lymphatic drainage of his legs, caused his feet to be huge and ungainly. He wore no shoes because there are no shoes I have ever seen that could cover those horrid feet. They appeared hideously large, like clown feet at the circus, and he could walk only by markedly flexing his hips and raising his knees high into the air. This motion caused him to waddle from side to side, making the whole scene all the more grotesque. He did not seem unhappy, but I could not bring myself to photograph him.

Laborers employed as cutters to make marble trays inlaid with semiprecious stones for the tourists work in sweatshops where they sit on the floor with poor lighting conditions and are paid about 1,000 rupees per month (about thirty dollars at the time) for working ten to twelve hours a day.

As I observed all of this, it made me ask how my Christian beliefs that I had acquired and formulated in the modern West were different from the values and mores of the millions of inhabitants of the rest of the world who did not share my understanding of the ways of birth and suffering, of illness and death.

Faith and Grace

Acceptance of a moral code is not the foundation of Christian belief. The central tenet of the Christian faith is the acceptance of the grace of God manifested in the sacrificial death of Jesus Christ. But what does it mean to accept Jesus Christ? If a Christian does a good deed for a non-Christian, and the non-Christian says, "This is a good man who is a man of God," does that constitute Christian faith? Consider the story of the centurion's servant who came to Jesus asking for help.[7] He said that his servant was at home paralyzed and suffering terribly, to which Jesus simply replied, "I will go and heal him." Then the centurion, knowing he was in the presence of God, told Jesus he was not worthy to have him under his roof. In one of the great statements of faith in all the Bible, the centurion said, "Lord, just say the word, and my servant will be healed," citing the fact that he was a soldier in command of many obedient men. When Jesus heard this, he was so impressed by the man's faith that he instructed him to return home, where he found that his servant had been healed.[8]

The centurion believed, and his servant was healed. We do not know exactly what he believed about the personhood and divinity of Jesus. Did his faith make him a Christian? Unless he believed that Jesus of Nazareth was the messiah sent by God to the people of Israel, we would probably not call him a covenantal Christian. Classically and traditionally, being a Christian means being "transformed," which is an active (not passive) process.[9] If I renew my mind and no longer conform to the pattern of this world, am I a Christian? Perhaps it is so, because no one but God can truly know what is in the mind of an individual. The Universalist argument (or universal reconciliation) is based on the premise that the gift of Jesus Christ through the grace of God is for all people, and that the Jews, as the people who gave us the historical Jesus, were a hope to the nations.[10]

The Great Commission[11] affirms the universal mission. The task of spreading the hope of the gospel is placed upon the Christian, not on the masses who have not heard it proclaimed. Those who are infused with the grace of God are obligated out of a sense of gratitude to do good works that glorify God in heaven:

"For we are God's workmanship, created in Jesus Christ to do good works, which God prepared in advance for us to do."[12] There is, however, no similar obligation for those who are the recipients of grace. We can only speculate about the responses of the centurion's servant, Jairus's daughter,[13] or those released from the tombs after the resurrection.[14] All of these people were the recipients of grace, but what did they believe? We have no indication what they did after they experienced these life-changing events.

If Jesus' death and resurrection atoned for all sin, and if not knowing about these events is a sin, then that sin was forgiven at the crucifixion. It might be a sin to know about the saving grace of the resurrection and not believe. This was C. S. Lewis's position against universalism in *The Great Divorce*,[15] although he was more certain about the consequences of conscious denial of the truth. This harsh absolutism leaves no room, however, for the skeptic or the doubter. Surely a loving and compassionate creator sitting in final judgment of those who doubt will give them the opportunity to see and believe before the judgment. Perhaps only those who see and no longer just doubt but actively choose to reject the truth are doomed. I cannot possibly know this. Those who have not seen or heard cannot be damned by a gracious, loving God, in my opinion, especially if their ignorance is caused by human folly, laziness, or corruption. Ultimately, I cannot know how God will judge, because only he can know.

The unpardonable sin[16] is blasphemy (rejection) against the Holy Spirit that requires a presupposed trinitarian comprehension of God. This sin can be committed only by those with an advanced understanding of the beautiful complexity of divine love and grace. Rejecting such wisdom, it seems to me, would be worthy of condemnation. Working actively for the destruction of truth (i.e., against grace) is an evil that involves plots against goodness and righteousness. It requires consciousness enslavement or self-enslavement of people along with willful acts to defile the name of God, to destroy other people, to violate freedom, to withhold love, or to deny justice. Without shame, regret, remorse, or contrition, these acts seem to me to border on being unpardonable but are not so, perhaps, unless one consciously denies God's grace in embracing them. Yet, I cannot know. If I say, "I know that God came to earth in the person of Jesus Christ, that he died for my sins and for the sins of the world, and that his grace is free and sufficient and requires no act on my part except the acceptance of the gift," then I believe and I am saved. If I then say, "Yet, I deny the love of God, I refuse to accept what God has done for me, I will follow all my desires without guilt or contrition, and I will abuse my fellow man to satisfy my wants and needs without regard to their needs; further, I deny what I know to be my obligation to humanity," then I possibly have committed the unpardonable sin. I leave this to God's wisdom and grace.

Short of this, because "all have sinned and fall short of the glory of God,"[17] even the believer cannot say that his belief has purchased his salvation. It is the death of Jesus Christ that has purchased it, and the believer enters the kingdom of God when he acknowledges this belief. For others, they enter the kingdom only after death because this is promised in the Scriptures.[18]

---

[1] Gätner, Otto. Baedeker's Athens. Translated by James Hogarth. Upper Saddle River, NJ: Prentice Hall Press, 1987.
[2] Acts 17:4
[3] Acts 17:16-20

4. Harris, Ralph W. (Executive Editor). *The New Testament Study Bible—Acts*. Springfield, MO: The Complete Biblical Library, 1991, 425.
5. Acts 17:20-31
6. Acts 22:4-10
7. Matthew 8:5-13
8. Ibid
9. "Do not conform any longer to the pattern of this world, but be transformed by the renewing of your mind.... Then you will be able to test and approve what God's will is—his good, pleasing and perfect will." Romans 12:2, 8
10. Matt 24:14
11. Matt 28:19,20
12. Ephes. 2:10
13. Mk 5:35-42
14. Matt 27:52,53
15. Lewis, C. S. *The Great Divorce*. New York: Simon and Schuster, 1996, 124.
16. Matt 12:31,32
17. Romans 3:23
18. Hebrews 11

13

A Christian Perspective on Suffering and Death

> The church cannot make the difficulty of reality less difficult. What I hope the church can do... is help us bear the difficulty without engaging in false hopes... Let us be a society that refuses to give easy answers to the difficulty of reality... whose members strive to tell one another the truth about the difficulties of reality.[1]
>
> —Stanley Hauerwas

Our response to suffering must be to love more perfectly, and to be in communion (i.e., mutual participation) with God. We are thereby open to the *veritas* that will be revealed.[2] Scientific truth comes not from a dissection of reality into unrelated parts, but from a mindful contemplation of the integrated, harmonious, and purposeful creation. A view of a creation without God that plummets randomly into an abyss of extinction can never be open to an enlightened order that will lead us out of our spiritual suffering in the midst of our physical pain.

How, then, are we to perceive suffering and death? Sadly (and I do mean sadly), many patients and their families have virtually no practical, firsthand knowledge about death before they confront their own illnesses.[3] They have formed their assumptions about death either through conjecture or the vicarious experience of the media. A few have used pure reason or reason combined with faith to consider death and ponder its depths. Considering death by reason alone, however, leads to the bleak conclusions of the existentialists who find no purpose in death apart from the prior accomplishments in the life of the deceased.[4] These depressing and gloomy conclusions are best discarded because they cannot be validated through experience. That is, the assertion that we die into nothingness is an untestable hypothesis.

It is not at all clear to me why so many of us are willing to accept pronouncements about the finitude of life and about the impossibility of life after death when these assumptions cannot be affirmed by actual experience. At the same time, we demand that the rest of what we learn be validated through the formal and informal testing processes that we acquire throughout our life events and experiences. This illogical paradox of pure reason in consideration of immortal life is a conundrum for many suffering patients. Their disregard for the possibility of life after death is not supported by the weight of the evidence as I understand it. Their misapplied conclusions are a manifestation of illogical thought that both scientists and believers alike oppose with great conviction. We must reaffirm, as did St. Thomas Aquinas, that the only requirement for making sense out of the world is to believe that God exists.[5]

What my patients fear most is judgment and damnation for the transgressions they perceive in their sinful lives. A belief in God is not accomplished through reason alone, because reason is based in the finite and the immediate. Although inductive reasoning is certainly possible and provable, it is rarely possible to induce logic from the finite that is generalizable to the infinite. Even the mathematics of the infinite cannot be observed in finite time. Indeed, our admittedly incomplete understanding of the infinite tells us that knowledge of the infinite is possible only through faith alone. It follows that the first step in conquering the painful reality of our suffering and death is to accept by faith that the infinite exists and that the infinite is the domain of almighty God. Through Jesus Christ, God transcended the infinite and visited the finite for the purpose of ushering mortal men and women into the infinite reality of his holy presence. This *mysterium tremendum*[6] is not the naive touchstone of the unexamined life but, rather, its opposite.

When I think about suffering deeply and for a long time, I must embrace faith when I finally and with utter exhaustion realize that all my human logic and all the logic of the thinkers throughout the centuries before me fails to discover a rational explanation for our pain. Even the profoundly depressed woman with a failed suicide attempt, the alcoholic, the drug abuser may ask the question, "Why do I behave in this way and cause my own pain?" with no apparent answer readily at hand. Paradoxically, pondering the consequences of the infinite has been a frequent activity of mathematicians and quantum physicists, many of whom now actively reject explanations of suffering based in arguments that begin with faith. In the hardness of our intellectualized hearts, we simply may be unable to contemplate an infinite creator who is willing to transcend time and space and, ultimately, to relieve our suffering.

The Meaning of Death

What is there to say about death that could bring comfort? For me, it is simply inconceivable that human life would not be immortal. That is my faith. Without immortality there would be no meaning in life for me, even in my few specific, willful, loving acts that I have done repeatedly over a very long time. Further, the fact that fear is a pervasive human emotion lends support to an argument in favor of immortality in this way: if nothingness follows life, as both the existentialist and the materialist scientist claim, there can be absolutely nothing to fear except the supposed meaninglessness of our temporal, earthly lives. But in immortality, all our fears are overcome, and nothingness is replaced by the all-encompassing, eternal love of God.[7] In death we achieve union with the one who made us, thereby conquering fear, separation, and nothingness with unity, love, salvation, and peace.

The fact of the historical Jesus[8] and the belief by so many in his mystical, spiritual reality leads one either to believe in God and immortality or to believe that humanity is afflicted with a severe and recurrent delusional psychosis tormenting those who believe in God. I have seen the reality of immortal life reflected in the eyes of patients who desperately seek a cure from fatal illness when they are outside communion with God. These patients know quietly, secretly, and silently that God is real, even when they will not acknowledge him. They continue to seek temporal, physical solutions in their search for the infinite. It is similarly reflected in the impatient acceptance of the gift of immortality by those who do believe in the certain assurances of their faith and suffer patiently, waiting for a physical cure.

The canons of the Christian belief in immortality are written in the Gospel of John.[9] The incarnation of God in the person of Jesus Christ is the most incredible reality of Christianity. Only when I grapple with this reality can I begin to comprehend how God can be personally and individually involved with my suffering, for I am created in the image of God, a little lower than the angels.[10] It is as difficult for me to accept intellectually the possibility of the resurrection of the dead as it was for those who first heard such pronouncements from witnesses who had seen the resurrected Christ. If we accept the possibility of life after death, our faith in that belief can be shaken by individuals who, themselves not believing, mount intellectual arguments against the plausibility of eternal life, raising in us a creeping self-doubt.[11]

St. Paul recounted to the disbelieving Corinthians accounts of the appearance of the risen Christ to Peter and the apostles and to 500 others. Despite this testimony, there were those who failed to believe. St. Paul understood that even eyewitness testimony would not convince the hardened intellectual Greek cynic of first-century Corinth, and knowing this, he appealed to the Corinthians' keenly developed sense of logic and reasoning.[12] He continued with parallel arguments about the universality of the resurrection by arguing that just as both sin and death come to humans through other humans, the resurrection came through the man Jesus. Only if we believe that God has dominion and power over all the forces of this earth can we believe that he can defeat "the last enemy," death.

How do we know that the dead are raised? We know by two mechanisms, says St. Paul: first is the evidential,[13] the written and spoken testimony from those who saw Christ raise the dead, and from those who witnessed the risen Christ himself. These first-person accounts are no less credible than the evidence we so willingly accept from historians who attest to the veracity of other events. The second mechanism is faith, "the confident assurance that something we want is going to happen even though we cannot see it ahead."[14]

We can certainly question whether those people Jesus raised from the dead were clinically dead. I cannot argue from scientific facts that we know they had died. The source of this questioning is our deep-rooted and fundamental skepticism about the ability of God to intervene miraculously in human events and in our personal lives.[15] Accepting that God could and does intervene in our suffering and death is a necessary and welcomed result of faith, and faith is a prerequisite to the belief that God can raise us from the dead. Our failure to believe in the resurrection of the dead is our failure to believe in God, and a god who cannot raise the dead is not God to me. Such a god is not worthy of my adoration and praise. According to St. Paul, if our faith in the conquering power of the resurrection is in vain, then surely we are fools and all of our labor and struggle is in vain. He argues, "[I]f the dead are not raised, let us eat and drink, for tomorrow we die."[16]

This creed, this way to live, remains the daily code for many individuals today who, in St. Paul's words, "are ignorant of God." This ignorance is held out as enlightenment among many of my former intellectual, academic colleagues and among modern-day existentialists who are too proud, too self-determined, or too disinterested to recognize a power far greater than themselves. I believe that this poisoning of logic and our rejection of the reality of the resurrection has led to our prevalent societal *ennui* as we have focused increasingly inward upon ourselves. It has led to the suffering of many of my patients who seek physical cures to spiritual questions. They embrace, for a time, our supposed and imagined abilities to combat our death anxieties with technology or with amusement and merriment until events in their lives force them to confront the realization that neither reasoning nor jocularity can deliver them ultimate comfort. Although I strive to deliver all the physical comfort that medicine can provide to my suffering patients, I encourage them to understand that it is in our embracing the inevitable reality of our deaths—along with the saving power of the resurrection—that we free ourselves to be fully human and relieve the torments in our suffering souls.

This reality runs counter to our intellectual reasoning and forces us to ask again a fundamental question that St. Paul asked rhetorically: "How are the dead raised? With what kind of body will they come?" This is a perfectly reasonable question for the intellectual, but it cannot be answered directly with data that can be examined in a manner that will satisfy accepted rules of science, forensics, and physical evidence or those of philosophical argument. It can be answered only by analogy, an acceptable rhetorical tool employed when teachers deal with an area unfamiliar to students. St. Paul responds with an agricultural analogy that the Corinthians were sure to understand, but only after he rebuked the intellectual inconsistency of their faithless questioning.[17]

What is so obvious for St. Paul is difficult for us to comprehend, that there is a *spiritual body*. Paul's belief in the reality of the spiritual body followed naturally from his first-century intellectual understanding that if there was a natural body, then there must be a spiritual body. For most of us, logic dictates that if there is a natural body, there *cannot* be a spiritual body! Perhaps this is not so unexpected in our society where personal freedom and individual rights have become more important than individual obligations and duties. A necessary consequence of doing as we please when we please is the requirement to remove the rules that paradoxically grant us our freedoms while limiting their unchecked exercise. To eliminate the rules, we eliminate the rule giver. In so doing, we also eliminate the possibility that a creator who demands obedience also could have provided the most loving solution to our most profound yearning that we would not die.

When we are too sophisticated to accept that we are both loved and saved from death, we need to be reminded that our salvation does not depend on our ability to bring it about. We are merely required to accept the fact that it has been secured for us. This is faith. The details of our salvation remain a mystery except that it has occurred through Jesus Christ. St. Paul tells us that we will all be changed in the mystery that changes the dead and raises them imperishable. The previously mortal body becomes immortal, and "Death [is] swallowed up in victory." We then ask with the ancients, "Where, O death, is your victory? Where, O death, is your sting?" St. Paul reassures us "[to] stand firm. Let nothing move you. Always give yourselves fully to the work of the Lord, because you know that your labor in the Lord is not in vain."[18]

A more difficult question with more profound implications is whether those who do not believe in the resurrection are raised from the dead. Historical church treatises argue that this is not possible.[19] It is faith alone, argued Martin Luther and others, that makes us share in Christ and all his benefits. We acknowledge that the origin of this faith is the Holy Spirit, but who, then, is responsible for those of little faith? Is it our own hardness of heart that prevents our receptiveness to the Holy Spirit, or is it a matter of God's election?[20] Logic would lead us to argue that we are created with a will that is free to choose between good and evil, right and wrong, salvation and damnation. If I choose evil and wrongdoing and reject the gift of my salvation, Christian tradition argues that this is a sin that will not be forgiven. Most Christian doctrines say that only those people who personally accept the gift of salvation given in the sacrificial death of Jesus Christ are truly forgiven; impenitent sinners are not.[21] This is an ancient mystery for which I would not presume to have a clear answer, but I believe it is possible that God, in his infinite, loving providence, may offer all of his children the opportunity to accept the grace of Jesus Christ until the moment of their death.

There are three reasons why I believe this:

(1) It is extremely rare in my clinical experience to observe those who are dying to be in a state of profound psychic or spiritual anguish. If they were facing bleak, uncertain infinitude (or worse, veritable nothingness), my expectation is that they would exhibit sheer terror. This has not been my clinical observation. I thus hold out the possibility of each dying person coming into the reality of the living God at the moment of death (simply through exhaustion of their stubborn intellectual defenses and the profound and persistent intervention of abiding, loving grace) and accepting the reality of the atoning death of Jesus Christ.

(2) If I believe in God and the death and resurrection of Jesus Christ, I must assert that God created us, that he loves us, and that we should thus love him. It is evident to me, however, that we do not all love God, and that our lack of love for the Creator is sin most simply defined. We avow,

nevertheless, that our Creator made allowances for our lack of love from the beginning of time.[22] He did not intend to craft a perfect creation, observe a flawed product, and then invent a solution to correct its inherent defects. The solution to the problem of sin was divined at the creation, and it is this salvation that comes to us personally and individually through God's prevenient grace. Yet, I must accept his grace and not reject it.

(3) Finally, faith and a belief in the forgiveness of sin and the resurrection of the dead are gifts, but our human arrogance leads some of us to reject them. Because they are gifts, salvation requires no action on our part for them to be given. We may choose to reject the gifts, but we cannot change the reality that they were offered. If I must perform some act or follow some ritual to receive a gift, then grace is not grace at all, but I must still have faith.[23] If God is love, he loves the entire human creation, but he created us free to reject his gift of salvation by grace manifested in the birth, death, and resurrection of Jesus Christ. Therefore, traditional and historical Christianity holds that we will not be saved if we obstinately reject the gift of forgiveness of our sins. When we accept the joy of our salvation, we are freed from fear and made free to love one another.

Some Thoughts on Suffering

My difficulty with pain and suffering lies in the paradoxical answer to my suffering that is, at the same time, so simple and so overwhelmingly complex that I am unable to accept it for what it is. We have become so desperately intellectual, so mindfully sophisticated that we are no longer able to become like children[24] and accept the solutions that are provided to us. In the simple faith of the child, we gain more understanding than in all the intricate schemes designed to master the universe through logic alone.

We who suffer must live confidently, then, while acting specifically. We all want to be loved, to feel valued, to be free from pain or anxiety, and to live without fear. As I wrote earlier, to live free of fear is to live in faith, to live believing that nothing in all creation will be able to separate us from the love of God that is in Christ Jesus our Lord.[25] Believing this, we live confidently.

To be loved in this life requires that we love other human beings. We are loved by God alone even when we do not love him, but his love is so profound and so transcends mortal time that few of us can be ushered into God's holy presence in this life. We are simply not up to the task. God has chosen instead to make his love manifest through the saints, through the priesthood of all believers. This plan fails miserably, however, "when the salt loses its saltiness,"[26] and we fall prey to the lazy narcissism of evil. It flourishes when we love one another. Human cynicism swells when we seek the love of God in others and find them wanting. We then soon find our faith in God to be wanting fulfillment. Perfect Christian love seeks to give freely without expecting love in return, but this is a most radical notion in our mechanistic, determinist, materialistic world.

This may suggest that our human failure is, in fact, a failure in the design of our world by God, and that would be so were it not for the incarnation and birth of Jesus Christ. In that act, God absolved humanity from the sole responsibility for failing to love or believe as he commanded, because in the life of Christ, he showed us how to love perfectly. To live and love specifically, we Christians can never be abstract; we cannot espouse merely what should be. Instead, we must abide in the kingdom as it is, loving others as he first loved us.[27]

Comfort to Those Who Grieve

Those who suffer, then—and more particularly, in my experience, the families of those who suffer—ask most expectantly why we must wait until after death to experience the eternal glory of God. I have found two answers to our longing. The first stems from the recognition that physical well-being is not necessarily the highest good, nor is suffering the greatest evil.[28] The highest good is to seek continually to abide with God in his kingdom. In fact, modern mystics claim that we need not bring about the kingdom of God; we need merely dwell in it with him.[29] The sad truth, though, is that most of us are simply too self-indulged to be able to inhabit the kingdom of God. We, in fact, do not need to wait, but we choose something less than God's perfection out of our fear, ignorance, and doubt.

The second reason why we, in our impatience, are not ushered immediately into the eternal kingdom is that it is our duty to wait expectantly for it to come.[30] Most of us, without having the awesome experience of personal suffering or suffering in the life of a loved one, would never allow the possibility for our concern to be centered outside ourselves. Faith is established most surely when there is nowhere else to turn but to the divine spiritual reality that is the living God. The recognition of an external force beyond our control that has the power to minister to us personally in our private suffering is a reality that many of us are not willing to grasp because it requires a measure of self-denial to which we are neither accustomed nor willing to take the risk of discovering. Yet, this is the essence of faith, the absence of which makes suffering almost incomprehensible.

---

1. Hauerwas, Stanley. *Approaching the End: Eschatological Reflections on Church, Politics, and Life.* Grand Rapids: W. B. Eerdmans, 2013, 157.
2. "Then you will know the truth, and the truth will set you free." (John 8:32)
3. See, for example, Nuland, Sherwin B. *How We Die.* New York: Alfred A. Knopf, 1994; Lynch, Thomas. *The Undertaking: Life Studies from the Dismal Trade.* New York: WW Norton, 1997.
4. Kierkegaard, Sören. *The Sickness unto Death.* Hong HV, Hong EH, eds. Princeton: Princeton University Press, 1980.

Existentialism insists on the transcendence of being with respect to existence and assumes a substitute for God. It also holds that human existence, posing itself as a problem, projects itself with absolute freedom, creating itself by itself, thus assuming to itself the function of God. This, I submit, is the foundation of modern deterministic materialism. It insists on the finitude of human existence and on the limits inherent in its possibilities of projection and choice. It thereby eliminates the possibility of immortality.

For Kierkegaard, there exists a gulf between God and man that faith alone can bridge. Kierkegaard insisted that religious truth is incapable of objective proof and can be appropriated only by an act of will. He maintained that ethics does not free humankind from dread and despair. We require a relationship with God founded on a commitment that has no conclusive evidence to recommend it. Faith is a risk, or a "wager," as Blaise Pascal put it. In *The Concept of Dread*, Kierkegaard described that the state of mind that makes freedom possible is dread. Through experiencing dread, we leap from innocence to sin, and, if we accept the challenge of Christianity, from guilt to faith.

5. Gilson E. *The Philosophy of St. Thomas* Aquinas. New York: Dorset Press, 1948.
6. This phrase is from Otto R. The idea of the holy: an inquiry into the non-rational factor in the idea of the divine and its relation to the rational. London: Oxford University Press, 1923.
7. John 14:2.
8. Theide CP, D'Ancona M. *Eyewitness to Jesus.* New York: Doubleday, 1996.
9. John 1:1–5: "In the beginning was the Word, and the Word was with God, and the Word was God. He was with God in the beginning. Through him all things were made; without him nothing was made that has been made. In him was life, and that life was the light of men. The light shines in the darkness, but the darkness has not understood it."
10. Hebrews 2:9
11. 1 Corinthians 15
12. 1 Cor 15:12-19: "But if it is preached that Christ has been raised from the dead, how can some of you say that there is no resurrection of the dead? If there is no resurrection of the dead, then not even Christ has been raised. And if Christ has not been raised, our preaching is useless and so is your faith. More than that, we are then found to be false witnesses about God, for we have testified about God that he raised Christ from the dead. But he did not raise him if in fact the dead are not raised. For if the dead are not raised, then Christ has not been raised either. And if Christ has not been raised, your faith is futile; you are still in your sins. Then those also who have fallen asleep in Christ are lost. If only for this life we have hope in Christ, we are to be pitied more than all men."
13. John 12:17, 21:14; Acts 3:15
14. Hebrews 11:1, 4; Matthew 9:18
15. Luke 16:31
16. 1 Cor 15:32
17. 1 Cor 15:37-44
18. 1 Corinthians 15:57-58
19. *The Heidelberg Catechism.* http://www.ccel.org/creeds/heidelberg-cat.html (Accessed September 13, 2014).

   Question 20. "Will all men, then, be saved through Christ as they became lost through Adam? Answer: No. Only those, who by true faith, are incorporated into him and accept his benefits." Jn 1:11-13; Rm 11:17-20; Heb 4:2, 10:39.

[20] Rm 8:29-30
[21] "For God so loved the world that he gave his one and only Son, that whoever believes in him shall not perish but have eternal life." John 3:16
[22] John 1:1-14
[23] Yancey P. *What's So Amazing about Grace?* Grand Rapids: Zondervan, 1997.
[24] Matthew 18:3
[25] Romans 8:38-39
[26] Matthew 5:13
[27] 1 John 4:19
[28] Merton T. *No Man Is an Island.* New York: Harcourt, Brace Jovanovich Publishers 1983.

> "Suffering, therefore, can only be consecrated to God by one who believes that Jesus is not dead. And it is of the very essence of Christianity to face suffering and death not because they are good, not because they have meaning, but because the Resurrection of Jesus has robbed them of their meaning" (p. 79).

> "Useless and hateful in itself, suffering without faith is a curse. A society whose whole idea is to eliminate suffering and bring all its members the greatest amount of comfort and pleasure is doomed to be destroyed. It does not understand that all evil is not necessarily to be avoided. Nor is suffering the only evil" (p. 83).

> "Physical evil is only to be regarded as a real evil insofar as it tends to ferment sin in our souls. That is why a Christian must seek in every way possible to relieve the sufferings of others... because they are occasions of sin" (p. 85).

[29] Westerhof JH. *Spiritual Life: The Foundation for Preaching and Teaching.* Louisville: Westminster John Knox Press, 1994.
[30] Psalm 40.

14

Lessons from My Patients: Grace Within Suffering

> We were promised sufferings. They were part of the program. We were even told, 'Blessed are they that mourn,' and I accept it. I've got nothing that I hadn't bargained for. Of course it is different when the thing happens to oneself, not to others, and in reality, not imagination.[1]
>
> —C. S. Lewis, *A Grief Observed*

It is often my task as a medical oncologist to tell a young woman with children, a husband, and a job that she will need four months of noxious chemotherapy to treat her early-stage breast cancer, treatment that will cause nausea, fatigue, and hair loss. None of these women has wept uncontrollably, although I have seen many tears. No one has cursed me, and no one has accused me of cruelty, insensitivity, or madness when I have felt that surely I must be mad to subject these beautiful people to such physical torment. I have told patients that we oncologists are an unusual group of physicians, because whereas most doctors make sick patients well, we oncologists take well people and make them sick when we give our chemotherapy for early cancer. Only three women in my thirty years of practice have rejected my recommendations for chemotherapy.

I have sometimes wondered if my patients have written my name on their personal list of the worst barbarians of the decade, but they never utter their dissatisfaction aloud. If I were deluded, I would conclude that all women with breast cancer are polite, schooled by their mothers, grandmothers, and aunts always to show respect to their physicians, but the malpractice crisis speaks against such trust and respect. I might conclude that nothing I tell them is shocking, offensive, or threatening, but logic says that is not so. They have, at times, asked me how I can see women and their families facing death regularly and repeatedly. These women have shown me grace in disfigurement, they face death without hysteria, and I marvel at their composure in the face of their suffering.

Sometimes I offer the cynical half-truth that I practice medical oncology so that I don't have to teach second grade, an occupation in which I could never summon the patience to face each morning and for which I do not have the requisite skill. I have told patients when they have asked why I treat breast cancer that it is so I don't have to practice cardiology and face death that often arrives suddenly and unexpectedly. I suspect that I could have been quite comfortable as a cardiologist, but my patients know that I am not sincere in that reply, either. The women for whom I care know, as I know, that I practice oncology because it is the most intimate of all the medical specialties, including obstetrics and gynecology. By comparison, there is great joy in obstetrics, and there surely is much privacy both violated and shared in gynecology. Only an oncologist knows the mystery, the completeness, and the personal involvement that comes in facing death regularly and repeatedly, whether death is conquered and forestalled temporarily or delayed for decades.

Letters To and From Patients

All doctors receive letters such as the one below from their patients from time to time. I am sure that my care is neither different nor better than that given by hundreds of physicians to their patients every day in America. This one simple touched my heart with its honesty and genuine gratitude:

> Doctor Vogel,
> Just wanted to write a little note to say thank you for all you have done for me. I'm not just talking about the medicine you prescribed, but for your personal input into my getting well. You're an amazing man and doctor, you are truly in your calling, for what you do is a calling of God and not just a profession. So many times I was in your office ready to just quit, but your encouragement and upbeat personality gave me new hope to continue. I don't know how it was that you were to be my doctor. I am believing it was an intervention of God that you are the man he decided I needed. You were always so patient and kind to me, even though I cried at every appointment. You weren't judgmental, nor were you condescending, but truly a gentleman. Never did you make me feel the lesser person, or a complainer, but you were always uplifting, upbeat, full of hope and success,

and this part of your personality flowed over to me, your patient. For that I will always be grateful. I never was a leader, always a follower, and I am truly blessed to have had you as my leader in this fight.

Thank you just doesn't seem like enough, so to you I say, "May the Lord bless you today and always as you carry on your quest to end this horrendous disease."

Thank you again,

[Signature]

I have also taken time occasionally to write to some of my patients or their families. When I learned that a dear woman I had cared for in another city had died soon after my departure, I sent this letter to her family:

Dear friends:

It was with great sadness that I learned recently of Judy's death. The memory of her and her life are a great delight to me...

[Just] as Stephen Vincent Benet wrote of Robert E. Lee at his death, I am certain that the winged claws [of death] got no groans from Judy [when they finally came]. She, like Lee, fought a battle she would not ultimately win, but she struggled valiantly with more grace and courage than I have yet seen in all the women with breast cancer I have cared for over the years. She was infused with life, and she packed more into her few decades than many women who have lived twice as long.

I don't remember that she ever complained to me about her cancer. She was so matter-of-fact about her illness, and she never let it get in the way of her living or doing the things she wanted to do. She obviously loved her job as a teacher, and I am certain that she was an inspiration to all of her students and colleagues as well. She taught them by example that courage, forbearance, and perseverance will overcome much in this life no matter how many or few years we are granted.

I was ennobled to have known her. She always brightened my day in the clinic, and I always felt that I got more from Judy than I ever gave to her. She was so special in that she brought joy and grace even while she was burdened with illness. It seemed to me that her breast cancer was more of an annoyance to her than a curse or a disability, and she certainly walked around it, figuratively and defiantly, so that it would not impede the things she wanted to do and counted most important.

She could only live in that way because of her abiding faith in God and her trust that things would work out for the best no matter what happened. She found opportunity even in calamity, and she showed all of us every day just how indomitable her spirit was. She had a strength of character that was vastly larger than her tiny frame, and a heart that filled the room. It was easy to love her, and I know that many, many people did.

I remember with some amusement her David versus Goliath battle with [her health insurer] and how confident she was in her [television] interview. I also remember her childlike delight when we got the insurer to allow her to receive [the drug they would not pay for]. It was quite a victory for Judy and for women with breast cancer.

I've missed her since I left, and I miss her even more now, knowing that I will not see her again in this life. I treasure her gifts of strength and beauty, and my faith tells me that all is well with Judy now.

God bless you all, and God bless the memory of Judy. I shall always cherish the time she allowed me to share with her.

Very sincerely,
Victor G. Vogel, MD

In my experience no one can endure a personal battle with death and not tell you all about who they are and what they believe. Conversations on an airplane or at an evening party cannot begin to probe the depths of what a woman truly knows and comes to believe in the way that discussing her breast cancer can. When a woman reluctantly acknowledges that death is more proximate and real than she has ever known before, our talk becomes very intimate. At times the realities of her disease overwhelm her with shock, frustration, grief, and apprehension so that she becomes psychologically frozen, disabled from uttering any emotion and incapable of expressing her thoughts coherently. Yet in these frightening and threatening times, I hear my patients expressing thoughtfulness and insight, their passionate hopes and fears flowing with clarity and understanding in the seclusion of our examining rooms. Sometimes I feel as if the breast cancer doesn't come with us into those rooms even when it is fully there for my examining hands to feel. The disease remains outside like "war lying on a causal sheaf of peace" so that my patient, unfettered by her physical concerns during our brief interlude, can embrace an opportunity of spiritual intimacy to delve into her most profound thoughts and hopes, her fears and joys.

These beautiful women startle me with their peace and grace, not always demanding relief from their physical agonies but instead yearning for a bit more time with their children and spouses, with beloved family and friends. Their disease brings their values into sharper focus, and they eagerly seek opportunities to travel, to wonder, and to dream. They look for time to be people who are more totally and completely alive. I tell my patients who have newly diagnosed breast cancer that with my treatments, I am trying to assure that they will not die of breast cancer. That is no small goal. When I am compelled to explain with great sadness to women with advanced disease that I cannot cure their breast cancer, they quietly and earnestly plead, often with little emotion, for just a bit more time, not for themselves but for those they love. They want to attend one more baptism, enjoy one more wedding, a high school graduation, or a final trip with a cherished husband. We would all want those things.

I suppose I could interpret the calm demeanor of these brave and beautiful women as weak resignation to an evil they should rail against more violently, but their quietude implies an enemy already conquered. Their calm belies courage instead of fear, revealing their certainty that the evil called breast cancer is already defeated. They live knowing that their greatest peace comes from loving those who are close by, and that in loving others, they quiet their own fears. I do not know if their serenity as they face death comes from the love they feel showered upon them from their families and friends, or whether they show love to others by simply abiding in the peace that comes to them through their certainty that they are deeply loved. The reason for their serenity does not matter, because they are tranquil in their blessings.

I cared for two women who both had advanced breast cancer and who both lost homes in the same flood. One of them had to move sixty miles away for seven months while her home was being repaired. The other lived in a FEMA trailer for two years because she was poor and had nowhere else to go. Both women had disease that disfigured their bodies and wracked them with pain. Both received chemotherapy for months that caused significant and disabling discomforts. One of them fractured her lower leg that was destroyed by her metastatic cancer. She required a metal rod to be inserted into the bone to stabilize it and allow her to walk again. The other had a tumor on her chest wall that ulcerated and bled. Neither of them ever uttered a word of complaint or anger to me. They simply joined me in a pact to do whatever we could to control their disease for as long as possible. They both showed grace and quiet courage. The husband of one of them described her as being whimsical to the end.

These soldiers know that although the pain and suffering induced by my treatments are not my primary objectives, their suffering is required temporarily because our adversary is sly and frequently lethal. He possesses real capability to wreck the utmost harm. We gather curious comfort, then, in knowing that noxious therapy is potent, and we hope that it will annihilate the feared and hated enemy. When I manage their nausea and fatigue, their lost hair and repressed libido, as well as their pain, I sometimes sadly feel as if nothing has changed since the middle of the nineteenth century when we performed amputation without anesthesia, when we used cauterization and leeches to effect our cures. Still, I see no terror in the eyes of my patients, not even among those who are dying. I often witness deep, mournful sadness over what is being lost, to be sure, but I more often see serenity and beauty, strength and peace as my patients endure their trials with quiet forbearance.

The strength of these suffering women does not arise from either weakness or stupidity. Stupidity would demand rapid and purposeful flight to denial, running unrestrained from the reality of their cancer diagnosis and the demands of its therapy. I see very few women running. Rarely, some women have walked away thoughtfully after measured contemplation in which they weighed a small risk of relapse in the distant future with the short-term suffering that comes from weeks or months of adjuvant chemotherapy. These women have judged my proposed therapy to be of insufficient benefit. Their decision reflects neither fear nor weakness but, rather, rational management in their minds of the risks they are facing.

I recall one woman in her seventies at the time of her diagnosis of breast cancer who declined my offer of chemotherapy after prolonged, thoughtful discussion with her family members. When she relapsed with metastatic disease in her bones nearly three years later, she neither cried nor screamed nor cursed. She did not accuse me of incompetence or of failing to inform her fully of her options or of failing to state my recommendations clearly. She made her choices, and she did not question me when the outcome was not the one either she or I had desired. She and her daughter did question me carefully about her recurrent breast cancer, the behavior of metastatic disease, and her prognosis. Never, however, did she weep or hurl accusations.

This is palpable courage. Such women face death knowing that their disease will ultimately conquer them physically, but they do not allow it to defeat them spiritually or psychologically. They continue to work and care for their families. They take vacations and visit relatives, and they care for those they love. They perceive clearly their looming fates, yet they do not despair.

I am amazed by this. Seeing these women teach school when their energy is depleted, travel when they are nauseated, and attend social gatherings without a hair on their heads both encourages and strengthens me. Their quiet confidence is not weak resignation, and it is not ignorance. I know they are not uninformed, because I have helped with their education about the enemy within. They ask me what will become of them and I say this:

> "Your breast cancer has spread to your lungs, your liver, and your bones. You are having shortness of breath because the cancer cells are causing your immune system to produce both fluid and defensive attacker cells that are trying to eliminate the cancer cells. The fluid is filling your chest cavity, impairing the expansion of your lungs when your diaphragm moves. A similar process is occurring in your abdomen, causing it to swell. I am hoping that the chemotherapy [or hormonal therapy, or both] that I give you will stop the growth of these breast cancer cells and halt the production of the fluid. I believe your abdomen will get smaller, your coughing and shortness of breath will improve, and you will feel better for a time. I believe I can control your disease for as long as several (or even many) months, but I cannot cure your breast cancer. I am very sorry that no one can."

DOCTOR, WHAT IF IT WERE YOUR MOTHER?

The response I hear is virtually always affirmative, reflecting a sense that my patients will do what needs to be done. Again, this is not resignation but courage, and I believe that it comes to many women from a securely held knowledge that God is present in their suffering. A rare few do pessimistically resign themselves to defeat, to living their last days in gloom and depressed resignation, but this is an uncommon occurrence in my experience. I believe these women know deeply and fundamentally that God is with them. He is participating in their grief and loss, and he knows intimately both their physical and psychological agony. He knows their fear of disfigurement and loss of beauty, and their fear of being abandoned for losing their attractiveness and their sexuality in a culture that cherishes both of these idols. He aches with them as he bears their fear of loneliness that comes when families are separated by distance or emotional estrangement during their illness.

Some of these women tell me that they know God is with them. They profess this belief with an assured confidence that is as certain as the realities of their diagnoses and the supporting presence of their family and loved ones. My patients have a serene beauty, a loveliness that perfuses them with stern courage, enabling them to face dangers with quiet fortitude that comes from knowing how deeply they are loved by God who made them, who knew them before he formed them in their mothers' wombs.

The husband of a breast cancer survivor took a photograph of me standing with her at a public fund-raising event. I am wearing a business suit and she, a sexy and attractive evening dress. Her eyes sparkle with the joy and knowledge that she has overcome her adversary. Above those radiant eyes and a smile that projects pure joy is a head as hairless as a cue ball. She shows not a hint of shame, no inkling of self-pity or self-consciousness. She walked among the guests at the soiree with great comfort, feeling self-assured but never haughty. I marveled at her grace as I observed her talking comfortably with all whom she met. She put others at ease, and I relished her strength as a silent soldier who exuded beauty through her graceful eyes that shined beneath her bald scalp assaulted by chemotherapy.

Where and how does such peace arise? Such deep beauty comes from knowing that in God's world, even breast cancer cannot own us.[2] It comes from knowing that God is suffering with us, that he knows all our personal tribulations. We can feel no loss, no pain, and no grief that he does not know or has not known. My patients are sure of this despite chests that no longer bear the breasts that long ago were amputated in our attempt to control their disease. Surely these women feel their physical losses. They know that breasts are important as a source of affection and admiration, of longing and pleasure for them and for their mates. They know, too, that breasts do not—cannot—define who or what women are. Breasts are nurturing, they are attractive, and they are comforting and sensuous, but they are not "woman." A woman is so much more profound and complex, so deeply and satisfyingly intricate, that a mere breast cannot capture her essence. Although our culture worships breasts, glorifies and idolizes them, my patients have learned that they are not merely their breasts. Her physical appearance alone does not determine my patient's beauty. She knows that her beauty springs from deep within, from a spiritual oneness with her creator. Her beauty rushes forth from a soul made and possessed by God who knows the profound and lasting beauty that exudes even from a bare, scarred chest and a heart that leaps with a joy for life that remains a precious gift.

This deep beauty breaks forth without restraint and knows that we simply cannot be separated from God's love for us.[3] Surgery and disfigurement cannot separate us. Chemotherapy and hair loss cannot. Knowledge of his abiding presence imparts this joy, and courage follows closely behind.[4]

Marilyn Webb, in her book *The Good Death*,[5] says that the good deaths she has seen or learned about have these things in common:

1. Open, ongoing communication [between doctor, patient, and family]
2. Preservation of the patient's decision-making power
3. Sophisticated symptom control [e.g., pain, nausea, insomnia]
4. Limits set on excessive treatment
5. A focus on preserving patient quality of life
6. Emotional support
7. Financial support
8. Family support
9. Spiritual support
10. The patient is not abandoned by medical staff even when curative treatment is no longer required.

Although I cannot ease all the suffering that breast cancer asks my patients to endure, I try to attend to the items on that list that I can control or facilitate. Indeed, some of my therapies themselves inflict the very suffering I am trying to avert, but grace and beauty abound. I see miraculous courage every day in the women I treat, and I continue to be surprised at the strength that comes through their faith.

1. Lewis C. S. *A Grief Observed.* New York: Harper Collins, 2001.
2. See the Jim Volvano speech at the ESPY Awards on March 4, 1993, where he said, "Cancer can take away all of my physical abilities. It cannot touch my mind, it cannot touch my heart, and it cannot touch my soul. And those three things are going to carry on forever. I thank you and God bless you all." http://www.jimmyv.org/about-us/remembering-jim/jimmy-v-espy-awards-speech/ (Accessed September 13, 2014).
3. "Who shall separate us from the love of Christ? Shall trouble or hardship or persecution or famine or nakedness or danger or sword? As it is written:

   'For your sake we face death all day long; we are considered as sheep to be slaughtered.'

   No, in all these things we are more than conquerors through him who loved us. For I am convinced that neither death nor life, neither angels nor demons, neither the present nor the future, nor any powers, neither height nor depth, nor anything else in all creation, will be able to separate us from the love of God that is in Christ Jesus our Lord." (Romans 8:35–39)
4. "Therefore, since we have been justified through faith, we have peace with God through our Lord Jesus Christ, through whom we have gained access by faith into this grace in which we now stand. And we rejoice in the hope of the glory of God. Not only so, but we also rejoice in our sufferings, because we know that suffering produces perseverance; perseverance, character; and character, hope. And hope does not disappoint us, because God has poured out his love into our hearts by the Holy Spirit, whom he has given us." (Romans 5:1–5)
5. Webb, Marilyn. *The Good Death—The New American Search to Reshape the End of Life.* New York: Bantam Books, 1997.

15

Resolving Grief through Service to Others

Am I a soldier of the cross, a follower of the lamb? And shall I fear to own his cause, or blush to speak his name? Must I be carried to the skies on flowery beds of ease? While others fought to win the prize, and sailed through bloody seas?[1]
—Isaac Watts, "Am I a Soldier of the Cross?"

"Let's build a church in the jungle of Central America." The resolution of my grief after my mother's death would come a month after she died during a mission trip to Belize that I made with a group of loving Christian friends from our Methodist church in Houston.

The Mayan civilization spread into the area of Belize between 1500 BC and AD 300 and flourished until about AD 1000. European contact began in 1502 when Columbus sailed along the coast. The first recorded European settlement was begun by shipwrecked English seamen in 1638. Over the next 150 years, more English settlements were established. This period also was marked by piracy, indiscriminate logging, and sporadic attacks by Indians and neighboring Spanish settlements.

Great Britain first sent an official representative to the area in the late eighteenth century, but Belize was not formally termed the "Colony of British Honduras" until 1840. It became a crown colony in 1862. Subsequently, several constitutional changes were enacted to expand representative government. Full internal self-government under a ministerial system was granted in 1964. The official name of the territory was changed from British Honduras to Belize in 1973, and full independence was granted in 1981.

Belize is the most sparsely populated nation in Central America. Slightly more than half of the people live in six urban areas, primarily along the coast. The various Native American groups living there still speak their original languages, and an English Creole dialect, similar to the Creole dialects of the English-speaking Caribbean islands, is spoken by most. In 1990, about 60 percent of the population was Roman Catholic; the Anglican Church and Protestant Christian groups accounted for most of the remaining 40 percent. Mennonite settlers numbered about 7,400.[2]

Belize remains a tiny country of just over 324,000 inhabitants in 2012, with a total land area slightly larger than Massachusetts. Life expectancy at birth is only sixty-eight years, nearly two decades less than in the United States. Somewhat surprisingly, the literacy rate among young and old, male and female, is reported to be 75 percent, probably attributable to the country's British heritage and school system. Only 52,000 people worked in Belize during the year before our trip, and the economy was based primarily on agriculture, agro-based industry, and merchandising. Tourism and construction were assuming increasing importance during the 1980s; agriculture, however, accounted for about 30 percent of a gross domestic product (GDP) that was only $373 million in 1990 and provided 75 percent of export earnings from fishing, forestry, sugarcane, bananas, coca, and citrus fruits, with an expanding output of lumber and cultured shrimp. Belize remained, nevertheless, a net importer of basic foods. (The Belizean GDP is smaller than the annual budget of any of the universities in which I have worked during my career.)

These difficult social and economic circumstances made it challenging for the local economy to support construction of a church building. The United Methodist Church, as part of its international mission project, coordinates and dispatches mission construction teams to sites around the world that are in need of new facilities: church buildings, schools, and clinics. The small wooden structure that housed the Forest Home church four miles outside Punta Gorda was badly in need of repair after decades of weather and termite damage. The South Texas Conference sent ten teams to build a reinforced cinder-block-and-concrete sanctuary to replace the decaying church. We were the sixth team, sent to lay cinder blocks over reinforcing rods and fill them with concrete to create solid walls. There was a grammar school next to the church, and both church and school served the rural community. The five work crews before us had cleared the construction site, leveled the ground, dug and poured the foundation footers, and laid the first three courses of blocks for the simple rectangular building.

Our emotions on the morning of our departure from Houston were a mixture of anticipation and excitement, concern and wonder, love and fear. We were about to travel 1,100 miles to work for a week doing physical labor in the tropics to the glory of God. The planning took weeks, and it had been carefully done. There were evening meetings at the church to acquaint us with the work site, the building plan, and the goals of the trip. The team leaders made great efforts to assure that no one would have unrealistic expectations of the trip. We were cautioned not to come with personal agendas about how the building should be constructed, and the organizers admonished us to temper our egos and respect the opinions of the other team members.

Our Flights to Belize

The Continental Airlines flight from Houston to Merida, Mexico and the Licenciado Manuel Crecencio Rejon Internationale airport showed us that there was little doubt we were outside the United States. Small stucco houses with tin or wooden roofs lined dirt streets and crowded the approach path to the runway. The contrast to our suburban west Houston neighborhood we had left four hours earlier seized us with silence. We departed Manuel Crecencio for the flight to Belize City with a short fifty-minute flying time. A surly customs official greeted us, and a second officer rolled his eyes when we told him our destination was Punta Gorda. Despite the official's diffidence, the city's web site says, "Punta Gorda is the gateway to everything from off-shore fishing, to river trips, as well as caving, birding and Maya archaeological sites. Not to mention, some of the nicest people you'll ever meet."[3] We were about to learn how true this was.

Belize is not a country blessed with progressive airports. In 1991, there were only forty-two in the entire nation, and only thirty-two were considered usable. More telling is the fact that only *three* of the airports listed the runways as having a permanent surface. Consequently, getting from Belize City to Punta Gorda was no simple task. Punta Gorda is a coastal fishing village on the Bay of Amatique, lying where the Central American coastline turns abruptly from the flat terrain at the Gulf of Honduras to run east–west along the northern border of that country. The Sierra de Santa Cruz Mountains rise to nearly 4,400 feet across the Bay of Amatique and can be seen for miles when approaching by air from the north. Because of these prominent landmarks, the destination is easy to find if you can see where you are going; in the clouds, the journey is treacherous.

The Britten Norman Islander we would fly is an ideal airplane for operating out of unimproved airstrips in the tropics. Its fixed landing gear reduces maintenance costs and makes gear-up landing accidents an impossibility. The high-wing design keeps the propeller blades clear of both gravel and debris invariably found on poorly maintained asphalt runways. After a Boeing 727, however, the Islander's physical presence on the ramp was hardly imposing. Our team chattered nervously about the trip in "the little plane," and they voiced some real reluctance to chance a flight with a foreign pilot flying under certification procedures that the group was sure were less stringent than those of the United States Federal Aviation Administration.[4]

The Islander had only one pilot, and because I was also a licensed pilot, I was elected by my traveling companions to sit in the unoccupied copilot's seat. We accelerated slowly to rotation speed in the heat, and we climbed out slowly. After passing 1,000 feet, the pilot pulled the throttles back after using full power for takeoff. I was relieved we still had two engines turning. *The pilot must have flown this route hundreds of times,* I told myself. *Of course he doesn't need radio navigation. Besides, we are flying visually, and the landmarks below us are clearly visible.* I watched from my perch in the right front seat and waited and wondered. *Can I find the airport if I must?*

The appearance of the Maya Mountains to the right of the Islander's nose told us we had arrived in the Toledo district. I had not yet located the runway at Punta Gorda when the pilot pulled back the throttles and we began a gradual descent. With full flaps deployed, our descent was steep, but we floated in the ground effect before arriving firmly on the uneven asphalt of the sleepy little coastal town on the Caribbean coast that is Belize's eastern border. The mountains of Guatemala were visible to the south through the mist.

Punta Gorda

We disembarked from the Islander happy to have survived the trip and eager to get on with our mission, but confusion reigned on the ramp because no one seemed to know what was to happen next. Our group leader said that the project foreman, Duke Walker, was to meet us and drive us to the hotel, but it was not clear how this information had been obtained or whether Mr. Walker knew that we had arrived. It was uncomfortably hot on the asphalt in the midafternoon sun, and we yearned to find some sheltering shade. Someone announced that the hotel was only a ten-minute walk away and that Duke would bring our bags in the truck once he finally appeared.

Having no visible means of conveyance, we walked—walked in a town with dirt streets a thousand miles from home, a town without sidewalks or street signs, toward a hotel without an address facing a week ahead that would be filled with events that could not yet be known. We walked past ramshackle houses with dirt floors where near-naked, curious children played in grassless yards, fixing their piercing gazes on these intruders from the north. They did not speak, their large brown eyes filled with silent, unuttered questions about who we were and why we were here. Large dogs barked, and the smaller ones ran through the streets around us, as curious as the children but much less silent.

The houses surrounding the airport were small and scattered among the dense, tropical vegetation that included banana trees, poinsettias, and bougainvilleas. The streets had been paved once, but they were not well maintained. They were now a random assortment of sections of pavement alternating with densely packed dirt covered with embedded gravel and numerous potholes that filled with rainwater during frequent afternoon showers.

To our surprise, churches were numerous throughout the town, and some appeared prosperous and recently built. Mr. Wagner's hotel was more like a migrant camp than a tourist stop. It had a general store in its ground level that reminded me of my great-grandmother's country store at the foot of Blue Mountain in northeastern Pennsylvania. Mr. Wagner's place had wooden shelves stocked with gallon-sized glass jars that contained food and candy. He used an antiquated balance scale to weigh the desired quantities and poured them from the scale's tarnished metal pan into small paper bags that were wrinkled from prior use. Modest as it was, the store had one prized landmark: the cooler from which Mr. Wagner produced refreshing, nearly frozen, Coca-Colas on these hot, tropical afternoons.

The hotel was a three-story stucco building with a balcony surrounding the second floor. Jim Glenney (my bunkmate and our resident investment broker/financial planner) and I shared a subterranean room that was, quite literally, on the ground floor. The base of the window on the side wall was level with the asphalt outside. I wondered silently if strange and dangerous tropical critters might crawl in through the louvered shutters at night to inspect the foreign guests, bite us with xenophobic vengeance, and inflict us with an incurable tropical illness. A dim, bare bulb overhead glared at night. Mounted on the rear wall of the room, an oscillating fan provided the only relief from the sweltering afternoons and early evenings. The concrete floor was painted red, and the drab stucco walls bore an unappealing ochre hue. There were screens on the windows and the front door, and a rear door led to a large screened patio which, in turn, led to the locker room–style bathroom that had four curtained shower stalls and toilets in wooden cubicles. There was no carpeting, and the lighting was poor throughout. There were a half-dozen Adirondack-style chairs on the patio that was quite pleasant late in the evening when the sun was low and the heat less intense.

During our first day in town, we strolled about, getting our bearings and identifying common landmarks. The town municipal building was housed in a cinder-block structure next to the airport, and we ate our evening meal there on the first day. We had chicken that night as we did on many days and evenings during the next week. Women who were members of our host church cooked it with a coconut sauce whose flavor defined the cuisine for the entire week. They even added the coconut essence to our eggs at breakfast, a truly acquired taste.

Fitful Sleep

Before we learned about the challenges of building a church in the jungle, we became acquainted with the realities of tropical weather. Jim and I had spent a leisurely Sunday sharing a worship service with the church members whose building we had come to replace. We took a leisurely walk through the town, getting to know its inhabitants. We were eager to get started with our work on Monday, so we turned in early Sunday night. Jim and I had tried to sleep, but by midnight we were tossing and flopping in the heat while reviewing the events of our first day in the tropics: the airplane flight, the primitive airport, the modest hotel, our stroll through the town.

We were about to learn that Belizean thunderstorms come mostly at night after the sun's daytime heating ceases. As we rolled fitfully in our beds, we were interrupted by a flash outside, followed in a few seconds by the first of the thunderclaps. Within minutes the rain began, and the flashing and booming went on for nearly half an hour. The rain was heavy but not drenching.

I witnessed some thunderstorms in south Texas that dazzled me with their awesome, destructive power. One that spawned a tornado ripped through the West Houston Airport on a fine, early summer afternoon, peeled the top off a hangar as if it were a can of sardines, and turned a dozen airplanes into salvage parts in less than ten minutes. Another whistled through our residential neighborhood and emitted a ferocious microburst that dropped a live oak tree with a trunk two feet in diameter through the roof of a Texas-style ranch home while the terrified occupants huddled inside.

The thunderstorms of Belize made the Texas storms look like cheap party poppers.

At 2:20 a.m., I was literally lifted out of the bed by a crash of thunder that made me think for a passing moment that a truck had crashed into the front wall of the hotel. When my head cleared, I was aware of rain that sounded as if we were at the base of a waterfall. With each flash of lightning, the street outside was illuminated by bright daylight. The wind beat sheets of rain against the walls of the hotel and through the louvered windows. When it seemed that the rain could not possibly continue any longer, it stopped almost as abruptly as it had started. The thunder demon had stalked the night, grabbing our attention while both frightening us and reminding us of home.

Silence was all that we heard next—silence and the dripping of the water from the holes in the rainspouts. What we did not hear was the rhythmic oscillation of the wall fan that provided the only cooling in our steamy room. We tried the light, with no result. We thought that certainly the power would be restored in a short time, the way we were accustomed to it being restored at home. We waited and waited, tossing uncomfortably on damp sheets in the sweltering heat.

Flourishing in the Shade

The next morning, after a night of restless disquiet with no fan to provide relief, we learned that power is often not restored for many hours after a Belizean storm. This also meant there was no water for a shower because the water pump was electrically driven. We carried the night's perspiration with us to breakfast.

Our eagerness to begin working helped somewhat to ease our sticky, odorous discomfort, but not completely.

We walked to the dining shanty at the airport, and the morning breeze helped to refresh us somewhat. We ate a hearty breakfast of coconut milk–flavored scrambled eggs, bacon, toast, coffee, and juice. We had more passionate discussions about the coming workweek, and our eagerness to get on with the building project soon made us forget that we had not showered. We walked back to the hotel and piled into the back of a well-worn panel truck that carried both construction tools and the local masons with us along an unimproved dirt road to the construction site about 4 miles away. The ride was hot and bumpy, and it was difficult to remain seated upright as we pitched and rolled along the uneven road.

Upon our arrival at the work site, we were told by our foreman, Duke, that our job was not to lay block, but rather to assist the local masons who had been hired for the job of laying the block. Duke had remained at the construction site to provide continuity for the project, instructing each new group arriving weekly about the standard operating procedures. He had driven a van full of construction tools to the building site from south Texas before construction began. He recounted harrowing tales of passing through customs in both Mexico and Guatemala and of almost having the tools confiscated several times. He informed us that we, like all of the groups who came before us, were to be the "unskilled" labor, a role to which we professionals were unaccustomed. Other than summer work during high school and college, this was the first time in my life I had supplied unskilled labor.

We carried blocks to the masons each day and mixed mortar to keep them supplied, but the local masons were painfully slow, and we were irritated by their leisurely pace. We watched them standing in front of a wall in progress for minutes at a time without doing any visible work. They indulged in frequent breaks, and it often took them as long as fifteen minutes to lay a single block! They were obviously unaware of our personal timetable to complete the job.

Everything that happened at the construction site we did by hand. We sawed steel reinforcing rods ("rebar") by hand with hacksaws. We bent the rebar into ovals using a homemade jig and a large length of heavy-gauge pipe. We then tied the ovals to long pieces of rebar placed vertically in the holes in the blocks using pliers and soft, bare wire. The ovals tied small "flying buttresses" to the main walls providing lateral support. The engineers in the group declared the structure to be hurricane proof.

Mixing both mortar and concrete was a group effort that began by dumping bags of Portland cement on a four-foot square of plywood. We made a crater in the center of the pile so that it looked like a gigantic version of a fifth grader's volcano science project. We then added water we carried in buckets from the hand pump at the construction site to the cement and mixed it slowly with shovels. This required four or five of us mixing continuously for ten minutes while the masons checked the consistency of the mixture periodically throughout the process. After repeated testing they eventually announced that the mortar was suitable to their needs.

When making concrete, we added a bucket of gravel to the mortar mixture and turned it through with our shovels. I hated mixing concrete because it was heavy, hot, tiring work. Others long before us had apparently recognized the challenges of working in the jungle and had incorporated their knowledge into the flag of

Belize. It is blue with narrow red stripes along the top and bottom edges. Centered on the banner is a large white disk bearing a coat of arms that features a shield flanked by two workers in front of a mahogany tree with a scroll at the bottom bearing the motto *SUB UMBRA FLOREO* ("I Flourish in the Shade"). How appropriate for the exhausted North Americans!

When we finished the mixing, we filled five-gallon buckets half full (that was all we could carry) and lugged them to the rising walls. Using large, heavy plastic drinking cups that you find at sports stadiums and that we had brought with us in large quantities, we scooped the concrete from the buckets and poured it into the holes in the blocks. We had to do this as each course of blocks was laid so that the concrete could fall through and completely fill the hollow blocks. To eliminate the spaces in the blocks that were not filled with the first pour, we manually rammed a length of rebar into the holes in the blocks and through the concrete to distribute it evenly. It was slow, exhausting work as we scooped with the cup, poured concrete into the holes, and tamped the holes with the rebar.

A Necessary Siesta

Lunch each day was a relaxing break from the physical labor that was more intense than our usual daily sedentary routines at home. We ate in a springhouse, a small, breezy, open building behind the construction site, down the hill toward the school. The school itself consisted of two single-story stucco buildings with tile roofs placed at right angles to each other. The courtyard formed by their inner walls was a staging area with a flagpole where the students assembled before the start of classes each morning. Whether for our benefit or as a matter of routine, they sang lovely songs, the melodies rolling beautifully up the hill to the construction site as we began our workday. By the end of each morning, the cooks had prepared a hot meal that we served ourselves buffet-style. We sat on benches at wooden tables covered with oilskin tablecloths and ate chicken or turkey, ham or fish, mashed potatoes and fresh beans, cornbread and rolls, cake and Jell-O for desert. Our appetites were hardy because we were burning a colossal number of calories, even in the jungle's heat.

On most days, we used the time after lunch for a genuine tropical siesta. The short nap revitalized us before we returned to the rigors of the afternoon's labors. By midweek, however, some of the more adventurous members of our team wanted to explore the jungle near the work site. They had heard that there was a graveyard nearby, and they thought it would be an exciting diversion to locate the graves and read some of the headstones. After one fine lunch, the adventurers set out in waist-high grass to find the hoped-for markers. They returned exhausted after thirty minutes of fruitless searching through the tall grass that created conditions like wading through deep snow.

One night at dinner at the end of the week, I got out the guidebook[5] to share with the group what I had learned about the wildlife of Belize. I discovered that the jungle was populated by a variety of interesting and dangerous species. One was named the "jumping Tommygoff," a particularly pesky tree snake that seemed to enjoy lying in wait on the boughs of jungle trees so that it could leap distances as long as ten feet and attach itself to the neck of its unsuspecting prey. The snake was reported to be tenacious in this activity and had the reputation of leaping without provocation upon targets substantially larger than itself. The "you don't bother it and it won't bother you" rule I had learned in the Boy Scouts did not apply here.

If that weren't menacing enough, there was also a reptile simply known locally as the "ten-minute snake." This little creature was reported to be only six inches long and was not nearly as aggressive as the Tommygoff. The problem was that you couldn't see it easily, and it had a penchant for biting to protect itself. Apparently, the snake was endowed with spectacular protection in the form of venom that was uniformly lethal within ten minutes of its bite. There was no known antidote, although it would scarcely matter if you got bitten in the jungle, thirty minutes or more from the nearest medical attention. As I read that information aloud from the guidebook that evening to my dinner mates, there was startled amazement that gave way to raucous laughter as the jungle adventurers contemplated what might have been their fate had they encountered any of these troublesome creatures. We also learned from one of the masons that there were leopards in the jungle. He supported his claim by proudly showing us photographs of a leopard he had shot himself.

At least you can see a leopard, I thought to myself, although I wasn't actually sure that was true if the spotted cat wanted to pounce on you from a tree limb. I was certain that I would probably never hear the cat before its attack.

We didn't venture back into the jungle on any more explorations after these revelations.

Our Daily Routine

Each workday consisted of rising at six o'clock, taking a shower to relieve the stickiness of sleeping in the un-air-conditioned swelter, and eating breakfast at the bungalow near the airport. We then returned to Mr. Wagner's hotel to fill three five-gallon, blaze orange plastic coolers with water from an ingeniously designed cistern that collected rainwater from the rainspouts that drained the hotel's roofs. The spouts all ran to a large, covered concrete vat. There was a spigot at the base of the vat that we used to fill the coolers. We then added plastic bags containing solid blocks of ice from Mr. Wagner's freezer that managed to keep the drinking water cold throughout the workday.

Duke assured us that the water was safe to drink. We regarded him as a healthy validation of this claim of safety because he had been drinking the water for weeks and had not once suffered any ill effects. He did warn us not to drink the water from the pump at the construction site because its microbiological status was in question. When I observed the cooks from the church using that water at the construction site, I was not reassured. They used it not only for cooking but also to make the instant punch we drank with our lunch each day. The punch, though, was not our largest potential dose of Belizean bacteria, because we drank only a few glasses with each meal. It was the water we drank from Mr. Wagner's cistern that was going to offer us the largest recurring dose of those pathogenic organisms because we drank it literally by the gallon. Each day we brought fifteen gallons to the work site; we seldom dumped out more than several quarts at the end of the day. During my first day on the job, I noted in my diary that I drank five quarts! I stopped counting on subsequent days, but a bout of "the trots" or "Montezuma's revenge" seemed inevitable given the quantities of water we regularly ingested.

Tropical Realities

There are myriad afflictions that can beset human beings who drink contaminated water, including typhoid fever and cholera, which can also be carried by contaminated vegetables and shellfish. *E. coli, Shigella* species, Calici virus and rotovirus, *Giardia lamblia, Yersinia enterocolitica,* and *Entamoeba histolytica* round out the dire list of possible pathogens. They all cause nasty, highly symptomatic clinical illnesses, but they can be controlled by proper sanitation procedures and by washing and cooking food thoroughly. Some are controlled by chlorination, but neither the water we drank from Mr. Wagner's cistern nor that from the pump at the work site was chlorinated. At the construction site, the latrine seemed to be far enough removed from the water pump, and the church pastor told us the water from the pump had been tested and was safe. We just were not sure.

During our trip to Punta Gorda, all ten of us eventually suffered from traveler's diarrhea. By day four of our trip, I had a vengeful case of this most feared of traveler's afflictions. I had no appetite for breakfast, and I was fatigued before I began working. I did not want to miss the workday completely by remaining at the hotel alone, mostly because I selfishly wanted to suffer in the company of others. There was some comfort in that. Nor did I want to appear to reject the hospitality of our hosts by appearing ill, but I felt so listless that I honestly did not know how I was going to work. I loaded myself with hefty doses of both Imodium and Pepto-Bismol I had brought with me for just this situation, although I had imagined I would be treating someone other than myself.

Diarrhea interferes with anyone's work, but when you are on a construction site in a jungle—and a coed construction site at that—there are some real and practical problems to face. First of all, diarrhea is dehydrating, and the therapy includes the need to consume large quantities of fluid. I was worried that the very water I should be drinking to avoid dehydration was the source of the problem, but I had few alternatives. Mr. Wagner did sell bottled juices and sodas, but it was impractical to carry gallons of these to the work site each day. Beer was out of the question. Chronic diarrhea is also fatiguing because of electrolyte depletion, but I could easily replete these simply by continuing to eat at each meal. There were, however, the practical problems of being able to access sanitary facilities in a timely manner. When those facilities consisted of a wooden "one-holer" to be used by twenty workers at the construction site, urgent access was going to be a challenge.

Boys Come to My Aid

I had brought a first aid kit with me that I constructed in Houston with both prescription and over-the-counter medications along with sterile needles and suture material in the event that someone slashed an extremity while doing the construction work. The boys from the school adjacent to the work site loved coming to the site to help us, as boys all over the world seem to enjoy doing. They came before and after class and would do virtually whatever we asked, all of them working in their bare feet. They pushed wheelbarrows, carried blocks and water, bent rebar, and made us laugh with their eagerness and enthusiasm. We had brought athletic T-shirts and plastic water bottles with athletic teams' logos with us that we left behind for the boys after our departure. They were delighted to get them.

When the boys learned that I was a physician, and that I had brought medical supplies with me, they began to hold a loosely organized "sick call" each morning before school. They presented me an assortment of scuffed and abraded toes and fingers that responded miraculously to alcohol sponges, iodine swabs, and a few Band-Aids. They began to call me "Doctor Vic," and they seemed to sense that I needed their help when I was in the throes of my bout of diarrhea. I am not sure why they were not in class that particular Wednesday morning, but three of them offered their help to move a truckload of blocks that had been unloaded in a corner of the construction site into the center of the church building. The temporary dirt floor of the new building was four or five feet above the lawn where the blocks had been deposited, too far away to be easily accessible to the masons. We needed to get the blocks closer.

The boys constructed a system of planks leading from the lawn across a pile of dirt in front of the building that was created when the foundation was excavated. From the top of the pile, another plank led across the threshold of what would eventually become the front doorway of the church. A final set of planks led from there into the center of the church building. The scaffolding for the masons was inside the walls, making the inside of the church the ideal place to pile the blocks for later distribution to the masons.

Together we devised a plan to move the cinder blocks. I sat on the piles of blocks outside the church because that was all I had the strength to do as I struggled with the ravages of my diarrhea. The boys were only eight or nine years old, in the third or fourth grade, and they couldn't have weighed more than fifty or sixty pounds each; the blocks weighed twelve pounds apiece. I helped them fill a wheelbarrow with three or four blocks, all that the boys could manage in a single load. With a running start, one of the boys was able to push the wheelbarrow up the incline and over the threshold of the doorway, with a willing helper running eagerly behind, both of them barefoot. Once inside, they somehow emptied the wheelbarrow, and the smaller of the boys pushed the barrow back on the return trip. Amazingly, I did not have to suture a single cut or remove a single shard of wire or wood from the feet of these delightful boys.

In six hours we moved hundreds of blocks across the planks that I called the "Highway to Heaven." I wondered what the Occupational Safety and Health Administration inspectors would have called it at an American work site, or how long the list of violations cited against us would have been for endangering these minors in such hazardous work. I certainly was concerned about their safety, but I was not about to deny their offer to help. They giggled with energized excitement as they all eagerly helped with the work. It seemed inappropriate to banish them from building their own church, and I was captivated by their eagerness and delight in performing the work. Those boys got me through that long, difficult day, and we moved a prodigious pile of blocks in the process.

A Night of Insight

My exhaustion at the end of the day was no better than it had been in the morning, but it was not much worse either. I didn't eat much dinner that evening, although I was able to control the trips to the bathroom with large and continuing doses of Imodium and Pepto-Bismol. Unfortunately, sleep that night was interrupted often by both abdominal cramping and nausea. After my second trip to the bathroom in the small hours of the morning, I was led to pick up my Bible, and began reading Paul's second letter to the Corinthians. When Paul wrote this letter, he told them of the trials that he and Timothy had endured while in prison in western Asia Minor.[6] Paul explained that he and Timothy had felt the sentence of death in their hearts. In prison, Paul and Timothy were in great peril, and probably suffered physical torture as they spread the gospel. I suffered no such abuse at our work site in Belize, but the loss of my mother compelled me to reexamine my understanding of God's purpose in allowing physical death to take a loved one. Paul's explanation is that God allows physical death so that we might not rely on ourselves but on God who raises the dead.

Sitting on a wooden chair on a concrete hotel porch during that long, difficult night in Belize, I suddenly understood that I was asking myself the most profound questions about my faith. Did I really believe the message of the gospel in my heart, or was this merely a superficial intellectual and emotional exercise I had been living while life was unchallenging but that I simply could not embrace after my time of spiritual crisis following my mother's fatal illness? If I could not believe that the gospel truth was alive for my mother, then my entire faith experience was without credibility. Never before had I been so conflicted in my faith. Yet, what Paul wrote was as true now as then: if we are not tested even unto death, why would we even bother to believe in God? More important, if he could not raise the dead, why should we believe at all? The answer that came on that porch in the dark of the early morning in Central America was that God loved us enough to send his Son to be raised from the dead that we might believe in him, and that his grace is sufficient to meet every need, even the terrible void left by the loss of someone we dearly loved.

The rest of the week was a blessing of comfort and reassurance as my understanding of grace became more tangible to me, and my diarrhea suddenly resolved.

Each day as we finished work on the church in Forest Home, we assembled beneath a huge mango tree to await the van we rode back to the hotel. As we sat beneath the tree on our last day, reflecting on our accomplishments during the week, I was struck with the realization that I had learned one very important lesson: to be a true servant, I must be willing to sacrifice myself in the manner of the Savior, and that means surrendering my ego, my intellect, and my pride to the greater goals of love and service to those in greatest need. What I was totally unprepared to learn in the jungle was that in so doing, I received more than I gave away. In this tropical setting, remote and physically inaccessible, I had confronted a most profound truth: my fear was always that if I gave too much away, there would be none of me left to do the "great works" that I had laid out for myself to do. Now, sitting on a rough, unplaned plank thrown across two cinder blocks under a mango tree thousands of miles from the great institutions of learning that I revered so deeply, I encountered a truth I had read about since boyhood: that receiving was in giving, that one's life is found in giving it away.[7] In this I also found the antidote to the affliction described by former Yale chaplain William Sloan Coffin in his observation that "There is no smaller package in the whole wide world than a man all wrapped up in himself." It was a moment of profound revelation.

Epilogue

The following year, the *Texas Conference News* of the United Methodist Church reported that the Forest Home Methodist Church, Forest Home, Toledo District, Belize, was dedicated to the glory of God with representatives of the Texas Conference in attendance, including Duke Walker and others. Eight mission teams from the Texas Conference had built the church over the preceding year. In the dedication sermon, the Reverend Rick Goodrich said that the church was built not with bricks, mortar, and lumber but with love, and that the church was to be a sturdy reminder of the Texas Conference's commitment to Jesus' commandment "Love your neighbor as yourself."

Tourism is the number-one foreign-exchange earner in Belize, according to the United States Central Intelligence Agency.[8] The government's fiscal policies led to GDP growth averaging nearly 4 percent in 1999–2007. Oil discoveries in 2006 bolstered this growth. In January 2013, the government announced that it had reached a deal with creditors to restructure its $544 million commercial external debt. A key government objective remains the reduction of poverty and inequality with the help of international donors. Per capita annual income in Belize was $8,900 (US dollars) in 2012, but more than four out of ten people lived in poverty. It ranks 125th in the world in per capita annual income. The sizable trade deficit and heavy foreign debt burden continue to be major concerns.

---

[1] "Am I a Soldier of the Cross?" Isaac Watts, 1674–1748.
[2] US State Department Data, 1999.
[3] www.travelbelize.org/destinations/southern-belize/punta-gorda (Accessed September 13, 2014).
[4] Three years after we returned the US Department of Transportation cited nine countries whose seventeen airlines were banned from flying to the United States because their aviation regulations were too lax to guarantee acceptable pilot training and aircraft maintenance. Leading the list was Belize. Secretary of Transportation Federico Peña indicated that the ban did not necessarily mean the airlines were unsafe, but cautioned that "travelers should consider using US-flagged carriers and carriers of other countries that have adequate civil aviation safety oversight." [Houston *Chronicle* September 3, 1994]
[5] Mallan, C. *Belize Handbook*. Chico, CA: Moon Publications, 1991.
[6] 2 Corinthians 1:1–11.
[7] Matthew 16:25.
[8] https://www.cia.gov/library/publications/the-world-factbook/geos/bh.html. (Accessed September 13, 2014)

16

Some Thoughts on Grace

> Grace means undeserved kindness. It is the gift of God to man the moment he sees he is unworthy of God's favor.
> —Dwight L. Moody

I believe that what I experienced in Belize (both in terms of what the boys did during my brief illness and what I came to understand about my faith) was a tangible manifestation of God's ever-present grace.[1] We usually think about grace in terms of expected events that occur as blessings. Examples include the birth of a healthy child, the successful college matriculation, the long-anticipated job finally secured, the marriage that endures, or the revelation of knowledge sought and achieved through diligently applied research. More than this, though, grace is also concerned with what does not happen, and an old maxim says, "Coincidence is God's way of remaining anonymous." Consider, for example, the illness that does not occur, the disease that does not progress, or the death that is painless. These are examples of grace.

Grace has three qualities, in my experience: (1) it is prevenient; (2) it is always miraculous, but not always spectacular; and (3) it is, at times, the refiner's fire. Prevenient grace refers to that which comes before: it is preceding, expectant, and anticipatory. Grace was present before creation, before the fall of humankind into sin and suffering.[2] We take great comfort from this assurance of grace that is, and was, and will be ever present.

Second, grace is always miraculous, but it is not always spectacular. Grace works through the Holy Spirit in blessings known and unknown to us, but it is cheapened when we believe it is deserved. It is made miraculous when we recognize it truly as a gift. Whatever our situation in life, be it suffering or triumph, despair or joy, poverty or wealth, infirmity or strength, all are gifts from God, all is worthy of praise.[3] It is in our trials, however, that we have the greatest opportunity to share in God's grace, and we should not limit his grace by constraining him to the outcomes we dictate. The ultimate grace is that while we were yet sinners, Christ died for us.[4] This is amazing grace, and it is what I experienced in Belize.

Finally, grace can be the refiner's fire.[5] It is not surprising to me that we get ill; it is astonishing that we stay well given "the thousand natural shocks that flesh is heir to."[6] A patient of mine once told me the troubling fact that her breast cancer was the best thing that ever happened to her! When she lost her hair, she told me that she stopped relying on her beauty and began trusting God. When she became nauseated, she relied on God. Then, tragedy compounded tragedy and she lost her husband, but she trusted God, and remained joyous. This was grace at work—the real, visible, tangible grace of the refiner's fire.

Having been first saved by miraculous grace, we have the opportunity to be instruments of his grace in the lives we touch with our own. God is not limited to the grace that we manifestly display to others, but it may be the only grace that others ever realize. As I have reasoned, a mystery of this grace is that when I bear the burden of another, my own cross (e.g., suffering, grief, pain, sorrow) gets lighter.[7] This is a physical calculus that crucifies the intellect, but it frees us to enjoy more abundantly the grace of the living God. Consider, for example, the true happiness of a servant such as Mother Teresa. Knowing similar happiness ourselves, we can pour out God's grace to others in praise for God's gift to us.[8]

When we ask, "Where was God when tragedy came?" it is more a question about our spiritual receivers being turned off than it is a statement about God not transmitting a message of comfort to us. Grace abounds;[9] we have only to open our hearts to know it in our lives. It is in our very nature to be sinful, but we are commanded to take up our crosses and follow him.[10]

We ignore grace when we create a god of our own making, when we send God's lifeboat and rescue helicopter away empty in our time of crisis, stubbornly refusing to climb on board and be saved from the rising danger that surrounds us. We accuse God of being absent when we harden our own hearts, but fortunately, grace can work through the Holy Spirit in blessings both known and unknown to us. Rather than demanding and waiting for the puny grace of our idolatrous, manufactured puppet gods, having been first saved by miraculous grace, we have the opportunity to be God's instruments of grace in the lives we touch with our own. Consequently, we should not limit God's grace by constraining him to outcomes that we dictate.

Grace is cheapened when we believe that we deserve it. We accept it as miraculous when we recognize it as a gift. It is in our trials, in fact, that we have the greatest opportunity to see God's grace at work. Having survived our trials by grace, we have the extraordinary opportunity to show God's love to others thorough our deeds.[11] When we feed the hungry, clothe the naked, visit the imprisoned, heal the sick,[12] we are instruments of God's grace and love, to use St. Francis's term.

I have often contemplated the curious juxtaposition of the time I spent at the Johns Hopkins Oncology Center watching my mother die and those hours I spent in Belize resolving the realities of her death. I blame no one for her loss except our own self-centered human ignorance that will not allow us to see the solution to the problem of cancer that surely must be at hand if we would simply yield to God's grace that provides answers willingly when we let him enter our hearts and open our minds. The resources of the Oncology Center seemed to pale in comparison to that spiritual renewal I felt in the heat of the jungle.

The year my mother died had been filled with unforgettable experiences. These included a visit to the White House for tea with Barbara Bush, breakfast with Marilyn Quayle in Houston when she received an award from the American Association for Cancer Research, an appearance on the CBS news program *48 Hours*, and an interview on CNN, all related to my work in the battle against breast cancer. None of this seemed to matter under the mango tree in Belize, and none of these experiences had a spiritual effect on me that was as renewing or as healing as my simple work in the tropics serving those in need.

I believe that the source of much of our loneliness, our isolation, and ultimately our suffering is our own self-centeredness, what the Bible relates as our hardness of heart.[13] Interrelatedness and a restoration of right relationships are the ways out of our despondency. By bearing the burdens of others, we do more than sublimate our own concerns, do more than simply remove them from our consciousness. We actually transform our grief into hope by focusing our energies on the needs of others, and our grief becomes a gift to the sufferers—not a cynical, remorseful gift, but rather, an offering of true sacrificial concern.

How can grief be a gift? It is because it is given not as a burden to be relieved through supplication and imploring, but as surrender that can be cast off only by shouldering the weight of another's burden and making it our own. "His yoke is easy and his burden is light."[14] The paradox is that it is my burden that brings me down, but your burden lifts me up. Your burden uplifts me because it is not wholly mine, and I, thereby, achieve some lordship, some mastery over you, and, in the same process, over myself. On first examination this may seem unjust, yet this is a right relationship, because in the kingdom of God, the servant is greater than the master. I bolster my own self-worth by lovingly shouldering your burden, and in doing so, I share more completely in God's providential love for me.

But how can my acceptance of your burden lighten my load? A Christian mystic would say that it occurs as a great mystery that defies human explanation. A psychological explanation would appeal to a blunting of the personal passions that occurs when energies are redirected to the task of solving another's problems. Is there also a philosophical or rational and objective explanation of this seeming paradox? I believe there is.

First, my perception of suffering in another evokes the possibility that their pain might be greater than my own. This realization brings me selfish comfort. That is, knowing that others suffer more than I do lessens my own suffering in proportion to the degree that their suffering is greater than mine. Sadly, this is haughty, self-centered, and impersonal, but it is a place to start. Second, we labor under an obligation, a command to love one another.[15] By bearing the burden of another, I discharge my obligation to love and thereby fulfill a moral requirement; I complete my moral duty. In discharging this duty, I achieve relief from the weight of moral obligation and thereby relieve another personal burden by bringing comfort to myself. Third, my bearing the burden of another evokes gratitude toward God from me in recognizing that my burden is not as great as the burdens of those whom I serve, and gratitude is a soothing balm. In gratitude we realize our own self-worth, and the elevated self-esteem that results from this, is therapeutic for many of our ills.

It is quite rare for us to love one another as God loves us; that is, to do it first, knowing that we will not be loved in return. Our love is not *agape* (unconditional, sacrificial, or spiritual love) that loves first and expects no return. We prefer our love to be *eros* (Greek erotic or pedagogic love) in which we demand love in return, often beyond the extent to which we have first loved. When our *eros* stops loving us reciprocally, when we perceive our emotional withdrawals to be lagging behind our self-perceived "generous" deposits, our poor version of *eros* wanes, a love that was more "immature-os" than selfless *eros*. The same is true of our *filia* (Greek for "affectionate regard or friendship," the love for our brothers and sisters) in which we are eager to love when we anticipate love in return but are equally quick to condemn when our love of brothers and sisters—both those joined to us by blood and those in our social community—is not returned with a measure that we feel meets our preconceived and selfish expectations.

We love selfishly, all the while wishing that others loved us more perfectly, frustrated that they do not see our worth. This is one of the ways we suffer. Our selfishness blinds our eyes and hardens our hearts, and we are rare indeed when (if ever) we love with no expectation of love in return. We condemn our brothers instead of forgiving, and we soon tire of forgiving even when the act of forgiving eases our own burden.[16] After an act of forgiveness, who has the greater burden: the one who has forgiven or the one who is forgiven? I lighten my burden by giving away forgiveness (love) and expect nothing in return, but alas, this human gift is not perfect, because we delight in ourselves for being prideful givers, and we condemn our brother with the burden of guilt that we require of him as the recipient of our false generosity.

I believe, however, that we have opportunities to be, collectively and in our nature, innately just, and we seek to reward the generous among us. Knowing that there is reward for generosity, we seek to be generous. Our generous love is imperfect, however, because we seek, either consciously or unconsciously, some reward in return. Nevertheless, it is viciously cynical to reject this self-centered generosity even when our imperfect love seeks its own reward. Imperfect love is still love, and we must seek to share it wherever and whenever we can, always seeking the higher good of more perfect, selfless giving.

Why do we strive? What do we long for? Why do we admire those who achieve and push human performance to its physical and intellectual limits? It is because we know that our esteem for human achievement validates and actualizes ourselves as healers, achievers, performers, artists, teachers, and scientists. The same adulation comes to us when we provide for someone who cannot provide for himself. Thus, there are discernible mechanisms whereby sacrificial love can reap benefits for the giver. How, then, do these benefits lessen the burden of grief? How can they remove our profound feelings of loss and separation? Why do the feelings of beneficence and joy persist after the deed is completed? Can it be that enduring gratitude cancels grief even when the gratitude is not visible in any sense that endures? I cannot answer these questions mechanistically, but I do know by my own experiences that sacrificial love surely lessens the burden of grief.

There is merit in our imperfect gifts, and any act of self-sacrifice must not be shunned even when it derives from selfish motivations. We are not God, to be sure, but we are imitators of Christ[17] when we love with gifts that are materially selfless even when we demand an emotional reward, either actively or passively, from the recipients of our feigned generosity. A gift that is not purely selfless is still a gift. A physical gift of time, money, effort, or talent that is given with expectation of tangible reward is still a gift despite our knowledge that we will receive something in return. The giver of a philanthropic gift receives adulation for her generosity. Those who donate time are praised as community leaders. Similarly, the mourner can expect to receive a lessening of her grief with her act of giving to others to ease their suffering.

---

[1] My daughter Heather told me as a middle schooler that the word *grace* is an acronym: "<u>G</u>od's <u>r</u>iches <u>a</u>t <u>C</u>hrist's <u>e</u>xpense." The Greek word χαριζ (charis) can be translated "grace, graciousness, kindness, goodwill; a gift, a favor; thanks, or gratitude." The English word typically refers to "the state of being protected or sanctified by God." It is no surprise that *grace* appears 157 times in the New Testament, and the Hebrew *chen* (grace, favor) appears 70 times in the Old Testament. The hymn "Amazing Grace" says, "'Twas grace that taught my heart to fear" in the sense of extreme reverence or awe.

2. "In the beginning was the Word, and the Word was with God, and the Word was God. He was with God in the beginning. The Word became flesh and made his dwelling among us. We have seen his glory, the glory of the One and Only, who came from the Father, full of grace and truth" (John 1:1, 2, 14).
3. In his famous poem "If," Rudyard Kipling captures the appropriate response to the life events he calls the "two imposters," Triumph and Disaster. Whatever our fate, God is with us, and the dogged persistence described by Kipling is, I believe, a manifestation of God's grace in our winning and in our defeats.
4. Romans 5:8.
5. Malachi 3:2–3.
6. Shakespeare, William. *Hamlet*, Act 3, Scene 1
7. Galatians 6:2.
8. Psalm 46:1.
9. 2 Corinthians 9:8.
10. The sting of death is sin, and the power of sin is the law. But thanks be to God! He gives us the victory through our Lord Jesus Christ. Therefore, my dear brothers, stand firm. Let nothing move you. Always give yourselves fully to the work of the Lord, because you know that your labor in the Lord is not in vain. 1 Corinthians 15:56–58
11. Is this faith alone sufficient? No. In the second chapter of the letter from James, the writer asks, "What good is it if a man claims to have faith but has no deeds?... Faith, by itself, if it is not accompanied by action, is dead. I will show you my faith by what I do... As the body without the spirit is dead, so faith without deeds is dead." (James 2:14, 17, 18, 26)
12. Matthew 25:34–40
13. σκληροκαρδια, (sklerocardia) is spiritual insensitivity or hostility toward God's revelation. It is used by Jesus in reference to the Law of Moses that permits divorce because of the Jew's stubborn unwillingness to accept God's plan for marriage (Matthew 19:8; Mark 10:5; Mark 16:14).
14. Matthew 11:30
15. John 13:34
16. Matt 18:21, 22
17. à Kempis, Thomas. *The Imitation of Christ*. New York: Book-of-the-Month Club, 1995.

17

The Spiritual Challenge of Sharing Bad News

Nothing in life is more wonderful than faith—the one great moving force which we can neither weigh in the balance nor test in the crucible.[1]

—W. Osler

What do I know personally about death as an oncologist who has been battling it for thirty years? I know that it hurts deeply, it robs us of life and opportunity and happiness, and it destroys families, futures, and promises. Paradoxically and ironically, although it fractures and ruptures, its effects are not permanent. In fact, death can instruct and lead to life changes that can even heal and mend, and death can resolve both conflict and dependency among those who mourn the loss of a loved one. It can actually create hope or make hope acceptable where only cynicism and doubt existed before. Walking through the valley of the shadow of death can bring insight and an inexplicable peace to a troubled and trying existence. We need to think more purposefully about controlling illness, without curing it, in the context of the everlasting promise of hope.

Advice from an Oncologist to the Dying

As difficult as it may be, accept pain and loss as a fact of life. Do not pretend that loss will not occur. When the time comes, let go of the dead, and surrender them to God. If you do not believe, or if you don't have faith in God, know that for the dead, the battle is over, their strife and suffering are ended. Remember this: it is as hard to prove the absence of eternal life as it is to prove its existence, so do not struggle with those imponderable questions if your faith does not allow you to do so. Honor the memory of those who have died; in your doing so, the deceased live on in eternity. Ask the "what if" questions: "How old would she be today? What would she be like? Would she like the new daughter-in-law?" Acknowledge life's stages and that we shall all pass through them, but that few individuals will be with us at all of the stages. We will have friends at school, professional colleagues, neighbors, and relatives. Sadly, the inevitable history of our families is that the generations pass away. We will say final and permanent good-byes many times in our lives.

We must make peace with death, knowing that, although it is painful now, the pain will lessen with time as the memories of the departed grow. We must replace ineffective technologies with caring and hopeful expectation for a better future or a blessed life in the world to come. We must become more rational by limiting testing and procedures that offer no benefit and do not improve the quality of our lives. We can mourn a death without becoming morose. It will always be true that if our lost loved one were here now to have her illness treated with the improved therapies of today, she might not have died, but that is the history of medicine and clinical science. Let go of regret. Celebrate the deceased, revel in their gifts, and forgive their trespasses. Forgiveness is one of the most liberating of all human acts. Even the passing of a hateful person with whom we had contentious dealings can lead to a lessening of our pain over time. Those who have faith will take comfort in the resurrection.

The questions below may be useful for patients, their families, and their caregivers as they deal with the symptoms and burdens of life-threatening illnesses and face the looming reality of approaching death.

What Patients Should Ask Their Doctors When They Face Serious Illness[2]

- Can my illness be cured?
- What will the time course be?
- What symptoms will I have?
- What will I be able to do?
- May I travel?
- What will it be like to die?
- May I die at home?
- What is my chance of being alive at one year with therapy? With the best supportive care or hospice?
- How much longer will I live with chemotherapy or other treatment?
- What effect will chemotherapy have on my quality of life?

- How likely is it that I will have symptoms such as mucositis, nausea and vomiting, hair loss, low white blood cell count, and increased risk of infection, and/or neuropathy?

Questions for the Patient to Ask Herself[3]

- Will this treatment prevent my death?
- What do I want to achieve with my doctor and with my treatment?
- How do I want to spend my time as I die?
- Will this treatment give me more time as I die?
- Where and how will I spend that time?
- What side effects might I expect?
- How much will it cost?
- Can my family afford this treatment?
- What would it mean if I did not get this treatment?
- What does treatment signify or mean to me? To my family?

What Patients Should Expect from Their Physicians as They Die

We doctors must be intentional in our conversations about the nature of the disease and its likely outcome. We must be both specific and honest in our disclosures about diagnosis and prognosis. Our conversations and treatments are not about winning or losing. Rather, they must be about what is truthful, rational, and realistic. It is neither rational nor compassionate to employ therapies that are known to be ineffective. Compassion entails being realistic and objective. Doing what might be effective or has a small chance of being effective is actually to test the natural history of the disease. I have sometimes referred to this as doing clinical research without a proper research protocol. We need to ask the very difficult question "Can we afford an increase of three to six weeks or months in disease-free survival if there is no decrease in mortality—that is, if this treatment cannot prevent my death, do we have infinite resources to expend on my care? How might our greed for futile treatments do harm to ourselves or others?"

ASCO recognizes the need for clinicians to address spiritual needs in the dying patient. I briefly summarize their recommendations here.[4]

- The goal of spiritual discussion is to elicit the spiritual concerns of the patient, family, and caregivers.
- Care team members must be prepared to address spiritual issues during the dying process.
- Clinicians should be adequately conversant in spiritual matters but should primarily listen.
- Appropriate referrals to a chaplain, pastor, or rabbi can be made when the patient is receptive to the idea.
- Care team members must approach a patient's religion or beliefs as a broad index of his spiritual orientation and make no assumptions.
- Spiritual resolution can be achieved by and among dying patients and their loved ones.

Communication with a dying patient requires the provision of accurate information, and its effectiveness is highly dependent upon the manner in which the information is presented. There should be a frank and open discussion of advanced care planning, advanced directives, and do-not-resuscitate orders. The doctor should inquire how much information the patient wants and should ask about the designation of health care proxies and powers of attorney. He should clarify how much information should be given to the patient's family. Although most existing guidelines for delivering bad news to patients and families do not have evidence from research studies to support their use, they are based on both accepted principles of communication and a consensus of expert opinions. They are useful measures to employ.[5]

Patients with cancer or other serious illnesses want to know certain and specific information about their disease, its treatment, and their prognosis. Specifically, they want to know how far advanced their disease is and how far it has spread, about the likelihood of cure, and how their treatment might affect their ability to carry on their usual social activities. Patients also want to know how their family and close friends might be affected by the disease and how they will care for themselves at home. Women with breast cancer want to know how their treatment will affect their feelings about their body and their sexual attractiveness. They want information about different types of treatment and the advantages and disadvantages of each one. Information about possible unpleasant side effects of treatment is always an important and understandable concern. Finally, they seek information about whether their children or other members of the family are now at risk of getting cancer themselves because of their own diagnosis.

Good communication requires a thorough assessment of a patient's and family's understanding of the course of the disease, the patient's capacity for decision making or the need for a surrogate decision maker, and the communication style of both the patient and the family. We doctors should ask the patient about her preferences for her care and her desire to preserve particular and specific aspects of her quality of life. Some physicians believe that an accurate prognosis will undermine the patient's hope, but available data do not support this conviction.[6] It is not at all surprising to recognize and acknowledge that patients do not want their doctors to lessen their hope, even at the end of life.[7]

Nevertheless, oncologists often do not give patients honest and truthful information about their prognosis and treatment options despite the fact that many patients say they want candid clinical information even if the outlook is poor.[8] Most cancer patients never receive information from their physicians about prognosis or even imminent death. Such lack of knowledge is associated with worse quality of care, worse quality of life for both the patient and their surviving caregivers. Although physicians sometimes limit prognostic information believing that less information will preserve hope, research shows no evidence that prognostic disclosure makes patients less hopeful.[9] Instead, disclosure of prognosis by the physician can support hope, even when the prognosis is poor.

For many doctors, communicating a realistic prognosis is an overwhelming task, and the prospect of providing spiritual care at the end of life presents a formidable challenge. Physicians are sometimes overly optimistic or provide too little information. It is also possible that patients may interpret what we tell them in an unreasonably optimistic way. Most patients believe that they will "beat the odds."[10] Published data show that patients who are overly optimistic often opt for more aggressive therapy despite the evidence that aggressive care is no better.[11]

When dealing with care at the end of life, we physicians must set realistic goals to relieve pain, to reduce stress, and to achieve closure of the patient's illness for them and their family. Families often believe that an accurate prognosis will reduce the patient's fighting spirit, but research shows this is not the case. Doctors must determine who should be told the prognosis and who should participate in the discussion about managing end-of-life issues. It is also important for the physician to grasp from the family what they already know.

Optimal cancer care at the end of life is a multidisciplinary task. To be able to converse meaningfully with patients about their beliefs and concerns, clinicians must themselves have contemplated the important spiritual and existential questions.[5] Our primary responsibility as oncologists is to guide the delivery of compassionate care. Patients are often forced, however, to confront questions they might prefer to ignore, such as the nature and purpose of suffering or the seeming injustice of a painful or premature death. These are ultimately spiritual questions, and good care of the spirit is essential to high-quality end-of-life care. ASCO recommends that physicians help patients in asking questions such as these:

- What is the meaning of life?
- Why am I here?
- What have I achieved in my life?
- How do I fit in the universe?
- What will happen to me after my death?

For most physicians, dealing with these questions will require that we refer the patient to a trained and competent spiritual resource such as a minister, pastor, chaplain, rabbi, or other religious professional.

After we communicate a realistic prognosis that is based in hope, we physicians must enlist the aid of the patient in her decision making. In a study of women with breast cancer conducted several years ago, researchers asked women about several important issues including their (1) preferences for various levels of participation in treatment decision making; (2) the extent to which they believed they had achieved their preferred levels of involvement in decision making; and (3) the ranking of their need for information and how these needs differed by age, race, extent of disease, and the types of treatment options available.[12] About one-fifth of women wanted to select their own cancer treatment, nearly half wanted to select their treatment collaboratively with their physicians, and a third wanted to delegate this responsibility to their physicians. Fewer than half the women believed they had achieved their preferred level of control in decision making, and the two most highly ranked types of information were related to knowing about the chances of cure and the spread of disease, i.e., prognosis. Perhaps not surprisingly, women younger than fifty years rated information about physical and sexual attractiveness as more important than did older women, and women older than seventy years rated information about self-care as more important than did younger women.

Families often assume that health care professionals will be able to introduce and discuss issues surrounding care of the spirit, but this is often not the case. We oncologists often lack specific training in end-of-life care, and we frequently report psychological burnout along with frustration and a sense of failure in our work. Researchers report that oncologists often cannot describe a clear method of transitioning their goals in care from treatment with curative intent to palliative care. In one study, a somewhat frustrated oncologist reported, "I felt more like a Rabbi... That was more how I helped than as an oncologist."[13] Experts say that oncologists without a clear method of communication can make few recommendations for palliative and supportive care to patients and their families. End-of-life discussions are processes that occur over a period of time as the disease process evolves. Palliative-care experts reassure us, however, that hope is maintained for patients with advanced cancer when their oncologists give them truthful prognostic and treatment information, even when the news is bad.[14]

A patient of mine identified with two separate cancers within two years illustrates this point very well. Mary was diagnosed with invasive breast cancer when she was sixty years old. She had left total mastectomy, and two of twenty-seven lymph nodes under her arm showed metastatic cancer. She came to me for her adjuvant chemotherapy soon after her surgery, and she enrolled in a research protocol, a clinical trial. She was treated with chemotherapy that we completed five months after her mastectomy. This treatment was followed by daily oral hormonal therapy. She also received post-mastectomy radiation therapy.

She was well for two years, during which time I saw her in follow-up every three to four months. She then developed symptoms of persistent indigestion. I ordered a CT scan that showed a mass just past her stomach, abutting her small intestine, that was obstructing both her common bile duct and her pancreatic duct (tubes or passages leading from her liver and pancreas into her small intestine). The mass extended from her pancreas into her duodenum (small bowel). A gastroenterologist did a biopsy through an endoscope that revealed poorly differentiated adenocarcinoma consistent with a new primary cancer (not her breast cancer) in her pancreas. He placed a metal stent in her duodenum to keep it open. Her stomach and a portion of her proximal small intestine were removed during an operation later that month, and we presented her case at our weekly gastrointestinal multidisciplinary conference. Doctors there recommended concurrent therapy with both radiation and chemotherapy. They all agreed that there was no intervention available to us to cure Mary of her second cancer.

I presented this treatment option to Mary, her husband, and their two sons. I made it very clear that her disease could not be cured with any known treatment, and that combined chemotherapy and radiation was likely to be associated with a number of side effects, including nausea and vomiting, weight loss, pain, possible bowel obstruction, and so on. After careful discussion of the risks and benefits, and a careful accounting of the side effects and toxicities, Mary and her family decided not to pursue the treatment. I referred her to our Palliative Medicine program, and we agreed that I would continue to see her every month along with the palliative-care team. We sent hospice nurses to her home twice a week. Three months later, she was using transdermal narcotics (skin patches) for pain. Her weight decreased during the following six months from 184 to 140 pounds, and her narcotic requirement continued to increase. She stayed in a hospital bed on the first floor of their home.

As she was dying at home, the palliative care physicians noted that Mary was sleeping more and experienced disorientation when she was awake. Her family and the hospice nurses observed restlessness, diminished sensation, and an inability for her to respond to stimuli, although Mary's ability to be aware of them remained intact. We gave her medications to relieve these symptoms, and her family was comfortable with the situation at home. The visiting nurses noted changes in her body temperatures, skin changes with mottling and blue discoloration, respiratory pattern changes, and an increase in her oral secretions. Our goal throughout her dying was to assure that Mary had a peaceful death. Her husband and sons—one of whom was a medical student—agreed with the plan that we had developed with Mary's full participation. She died quite peacefully after several weeks of care at home.

Receiving treatment to extend life rather than best supportive care has actually been shown to make a patient's quality of life worse rather than better.[15] Patients who recognize that their illness will result in their death are actually more likely to prefer symptom-directed care. Some patients (about one in six) who are aware that they are terminally ill, however, wish to receive life-extending care. Patients who report having discussed their wishes and life care with a physician are, indeed, more likely to receive care that is consistent with their preferences. Among patients who receive no life-extending measures, physical distress is actually reported to be lower among patients for whom such care is consistent with their preferences. Research shows that patients are more likely to attain their end-of-life care goals if their physicians are engaged in conversations with them about end-of-life care, and if the patients have a strong therapeutic alliance with their physicians.[16] This has certainly been my experience in my medical oncology career.

In addition, patients who receive life-extending therapy surprisingly do not live longer than patients who do not. Caregiver-rated quality-of-life and physical and psychological stress during the last week of life varies by the care that is preferred and received, and patients who receive life-extending care are known to experience greater physical and psychological stress and poorer quality of life regardless of their preferences. Among patients who receive life-prolonging care (despite a previously stated goal of minimizing suffering), there is greater distress and lower quality of life in the last week of life. This suggests that their primary goal of minimizing suffering was not met. Actually, most patients who prefer life-prolonging care ultimately do not receive such care during the last week of life in many clinical settings. Sadly, in fact, the majority of patients who receive life-extending measures have previously expressed a desire to receive symptom-directed care only. The burden of suffering experienced by these patients at the end of life is consequently high. Discussions to elicit the wishes of patients that are initiated by their physicians, therefore, have significant potential to reduce suffering at the end of life.

I have often said to patients and their families that treating chronic, incurable cancer is like opening a series of nested and painted Russian Matryoshka dolls as events appear to us slowly and progressively, one after another, over a period of time in a somewhat unpredictable manner and schedule. If an oncologist views his role primarily as a biomedical one, he will be more distant from the patient's family, often feeling a sense of failure and an absence of collegial support, with no clear method of communication. If, on the other hand, the oncologist views his role as being a guide and a resource for a patient and her family as they weigh their choices at the end of life, the patient will make better selections.

Drs. Tom Smith and Bruce Hillner (who are themselves medical oncologists) have suggested that there are a number of desirable changes that need to occur in the behavior of medical oncologists as we interact with our patients who have cancers that cannot be cured.[14] They urge us to stop doing laboratory testing or radiologic imaging where no benefit for such testing has been proven. They say that we should limit second and third treatments for metastatic cancer to single drugs rather than to combinations of drugs (because combinations are more expensive, more toxic, and offer little additional benefit over single cancer drugs given one at a time). They further recommend that we give chemotherapy only to patients with good performance status except for patients with cancers known to be highly responsive to therapy. I have told patients and their families on several occasions that if the patient cannot walk into my clinic, I will not treat them with chemotherapy.

Drs. Smith and Hillner also recommend that when patients are not responding to three consecutive, different types of chemotherapy, no additional chemotherapy should be given outside of a clinical trial (i.e., research study). That is, in such situations they and I believe that only investigational (experimental) treatment is appropriate. They further suggest that medical oncologists and their patients must recognize that the cost of cancer care is driven by what we agree to do or not do as we treat cancer that cannot be cured. They point out that both doctors and patients need to have more realistic expectations and that we need to integrate earlier and more frequent palliative care into our usual clinical cancer-care services. Finally, they say that both the medical oncology profession and our health care system in general need to perform more frequent cost-effectiveness analysis and place limits on care in situations where it is known to the ineffective or where the risks outweigh the benefits.

In my opinion, we certainly do not need either the feared "death panels" or a rationing of care. We simply need to have *better conversations* with our patients about what is both prudent and desirable along with what is realistic and possible. In a study of hospitalized patients with cancer in one institution, researchers found that the oncologist had initiated a discussion of advance directives that direct care at the end of life with very few patients. In a prospective, multicenter study of cancer patients, only a third of the patients and their families could recall having a discussion about impending death with the physician.[14] Oncologists often wait until symptoms appear or until they believe that nothing more can be done before they initiate these difficult discussions. In another study conducted two months before their death, half the patients with metastatic lung cancer had not had a discussion with their doctors about hospice care where the average length of stay in a hospice program for patients with lung cancer was only four days.[17]

Patients who have these admittedly difficult conversations with their oncologists experience less depression or anxiety, receive less aggressive end-of-life care, and rarely die in an intensive care unit or on a ventilator.[18] Moreover, these conversations allow the surviving family member who was the caregiver to have a better quality of life and would save our society millions of dollars were they to occur more regularly and frequently.

---

[1] Osler W. The faith that heals. *Br Med J* (18 June 1910) p. 1470.

[2] Westbrook CA. Ask an oncologist: honest answers to your cancer questions. *CreateSpace Independent Publishing Platform. www.createspace.com*, 2012 (Accessed September 13, 2014) Smith TJ, Dow LA, Virago E, Khatcheressian J, Lyckholm LJ, Matsuyama

R. Giving honest information to patients with advanced cancer maintains hope. *Oncology* 2010;24:521–525.

3. Novelli WD, Halvorson GC, Santa J. Recognizing an opinion: Findings from the IOM Evidence Communication Innovation Collaborative. *JAMA* 2012;25:1–2.

4. Abernethy AP, Kamal AH. "Palliative and end-of-life care" in Loprinzi CL (editor). ASCO-SEP: Medical oncology self-evaluation program, Third Edition. Alexandria, VA, American Society of Clinical Oncology. 2013;499–523.

5. Baile WF, Buckman R, Lenzi R, et al. SPIKES-a six-step protocol; for delivering bad news: application to the patient with cancer *Oncologist* 2000;5:302–311 Vaidya VU, Greenberg LW, Patel KM, et al. Teaching physicians how to break bad news: a 1-day workshop using standardized patients. *Archives of Pediatric and Adolescent Medicine* 1999;153:419–422.

6. Curtis JF, Patrick DL, Caldwell ES, et al. Why don't patients and physicians talk about end-of-life care? Barriers to communication for patients with acquired immunodeficiency syndrome and their physicians. *Archives of Internal Medicine* 2000;160:1690-1696 Knauft E, Neilsen EL, Engelberg RA, et al. Barriers and facilitators to end-of-life communication for patients with COPD. *Chest* 2005;127:2188-2196.

7. Heyland DK, Dodek P, Rocker G, et al. What matters most in end-of-life care: perceptions of seriously ill patients and their family members. *Canadian Medical Association Journal* 2006;174:627-633 Wenrich MD, Curtis JR, Ambrozy DA, et al. Dying patients' need for emotional support and personalized care from physicians: perspectives of patients with terminal illness, families, and health care providers. *Journal of Pain and Symptom Management* 2003;25:236-246.

8. Smith TJ, Dow LA, Virago E, et al. Ibid.

9. Mack JW, Wolfe J, Cook EF, et al: Hope and prognostic disclosure. *J Clin Oncol* 2007;25:5636-5642.

10. Thorne S, Hislop TG, Kuo M, et al. Hope and probability: patient perspectives of the meaning of numerical information in cancer communication. *Qualitative Health Research* 2006;16:318-336.

11. Weeks JC, Cook CF, O'Day SJ, et al. Relationship between cancer patients' predictions of prognosis and their treatment preferences. *JAMA* 1998;279:1709-1714.

12. Degner LF, Kristjanson, LJ, Bowman D, et al. Information needs and decisional preferences in women with breast cancer. *JAMA* 1997:277:1485-1492
13. Jackson VA, Mack J, Matsuyama R, et al. A qualitative study of oncologists' approaches to end-of-life care. *J Palliat Med* 2008;11:893-906. (page 897)
14. Smith TJ, Hillner BE. Bending the cost curve in cancer care. *N Engl J Med* 2011;364:2060-2065.
15. Mack JW, Weeks JC, Wright AW, et al. End-of-life discussions, goal attainment, and distress at the end of life: predictors and outcomes of receipt of care consistent with preferences. *J Clin Oncol* 2010;28:1203-1208.
16. Temel JS, Greer JA, Muzikansky A, et al. Early palliative care for patients with metastatic non–small-cell lung cancer. *N Engl J Med* 2010;363:733-742.
17. Huskamp HA, Keating NL, Malin JL, et al. Discussions with physicians about hospice among patients with metastatic lung cancer. *Arch Intern Med* 2009;169:954-62.
18. Zhang B, Wright AA, Huskamp HA, et al. Health care costs in the last week of life: associations with end-of-life conversations. *Arch Intern Med* 2009;169:480-488

18

Hope and Futility: What if it Were Your Mother?

> For in this hope we were saved. But hope that is seen is no hope at all. Who hopes for what they already have? But if we hope for what we do not yet have, we wait for it patiently.
> —Romans 8:24–25

If we are to make better decisions about treating serious and life-threatening illnesses, we must understand where we now spend money for our care, how our beliefs can influence our decisions for treatment, and why medical technology cannot cure all of our ills. I will review and discuss those issues in this chapter.

There is a great deal of waste in US health care expenditures. Categories of waste include failures of care delivery; failures of care coordination; administrative complexity; pricing failures; fraud and abuse in our health care system, and overtreatment (that includes, among other things, unwanted intensive care at the end of life for patients who prefer hospice and home care that represents hundreds of millions of dollars in wasteful spending every year).[1] We spend more on health care than the next ten biggest spenders combined: Japan, Germany, France, China, the United Kingdom, Italy, Canada, Brazil, Spain, and Australia. We spend almost as much in one week on health care as the $60 billion price tag for cleaning up after Hurricane Sandy.[2]

Annual direct costs for cancer care in the United States are projected to rise driven by increases in both the cost of therapy and the extent of care. In the United States, the sales of anticancer drugs are now second only to those of drugs for heart disease, and 70 percent of these sales come from products introduced since 2001. Most new cancer drugs are priced at $5,000 per month or more, and in many cases the cost-effectiveness ratios far exceed commonly accepted thresholds for medications used in clinical practice. This trend is not sustainable.[3]

Based on growth and aging of the US population, medical expenditures for cancer in the year 2020 are projected to reach at least $158 billion (in 2010 dollars)—an increase of 27 percent over 2010.[4] If newly developed tools for cancer diagnosis, treatment, and follow-up continue to be more expensive, medical expenditures for cancer could reach as high as $207 billion by 2020. In 2010, medical costs associated with cancer reached $124.6 billion, with the highest costs associated with breast cancer, colorectal cancer, lymphoma, lung cancer, and prostate cancer (see the table on the next page). The 2020 projections in the table assume a 5 percent increase in the initial costs of cancer treatment and in the costs during the last year of life.

Cost in US 2010 dollars, in billions[4]

Tumor site	2010 costs	2020 projections
Breast	$16.50	$25.64
Colorectal	$14.14	$20.39
Lung	$12.12	$18.84
Lymphoma	$12.14	$20.69
Prostate	$11.85	$19.02
Leukemia	$5.44	$9.35
Ovary	$5.12	$6.42
Brain	$4.47	$8.18
Bladder	$3.98	$5.71
Kidney	$3.80	$8.30
Head/Neck	$3.64	$5.46
Uterus	$2.62	$4.00
Melanoma	$2.36	$4.58
Pancreas	$2.27	$4.92
Stomach	$1.82	$2.88
Cervix	$1.55	$1.73
Esophagus	$1.33	$2.97
All sites	$124.57	$206.59

Assuming a 2 percent annual increase in medical costs in the initial and final phases of care, the projected 2020 costs increased to $173 billion.

Cancer care costs are divided into three important groups: one-fourth of cancer care costs are related to drugs, slightly more than half are for hospital care, and about one-fifth are attributable to physician charges.[5] Experts say that there are three means by which to lower total cancer care costs. One of the most important is reducing the amount spent for caring during the last month of life: 25 percent of Medicare costs occur in the last year, and 10 percent of the total Medicare budget is spent on care in the last month of life. Among patients older than sixty-five years, one in three die in a hospital, and only about half use hospice services.

Most clinicians will do what their patients ask. We have worked to eliminate paternalism in medicine, but in the process, we've engendered what ethicists have called "vending machine medicine," i.e., simply doing whatever patients request. Patients and their doctors have also substituted higher lines of treatment for thoughtful reflection and careful consideration of palliative care instead of therapy with curative intent. We have also substituted faith in treatment for faith in God. Our way of dealing with the unknown is to put our faith in the known commodity of medical treatment. Asking health care systems to provide feedback to practitioners about their overuse of care will help to reduce costs, but we physicians need to educate our patients to stop asking for things that do not improve their health in a valuable or meaningful way.

Sadly, physicians often do not recognize when patients are ready for hospice care. We clinicians need to educate our patients to ask for or demand palliative care when it is appropriate. In addition to all of this, we need to institute more rational pricing of our drugs. Patients need to ask about the cost of care and decline or not demand treatments with exorbitant pricing. For example, one single course of a breast cancer drug approved in 2013 cost $190,000 but does not result in a reduction in the risk of dying for patients with advanced breast cancer.[6] Another FDA-approved drug for advanced breast cancer that is quite expensive increases survival by an average of just over two months but does not reduce the chance of dying from the disease.[7]

I believe there are two reasons for our massive health care expenditures, most of which occur at the end of life. First, many of us live our lives in mortal fear of the inevitable, holding our hope only in our technologies and the perceived cures of our ills that will ultimately fail. Even professing and believing Christians often have not examined thoughtfully what they truly believe about death, resurrection, forgiveness and eternal life. The comforting reassurances of the gospel lead patients to make different choices at the end of life than those choices made by patients who believe that we die into nothingness or into judgment and damnation. Second, we doctors do an extremely poor job of communicating to our patients the realities of their projected and predictable outcomes and prognoses. We do not work with them to devise collaborative strategies at the end of their lives. We need to do a much better job of helping our patients frame realistic expectations.

We also need to do a much better job of securing advance directives that guide decisions at the end of life.[8] We need to educate patients more completely about following treatment pathways that will give guidance in settings where curative therapy is not available. This will also lead to greater patient participation in clinical research trials that ultimately help others. This is an opportunity for a final, altruistic gesture at the end of one's life. As others have advocated as well, I believe our national goal should be to have patients who have illnesses that will result in death participate earlier in palliative care and to plan their deaths at home rather than in the hospital. Better communication among physicians and their dying patients will help to promote and achieve all of these goals.

Victor G. Vogel, MD

Talking with Patients about Dying

Dr. Tom Smith and his colleagues at Johns Hopkins Medical School have done research on the ways doctors talk to their patients about dying.[9] I have known Dr. Smith for many years, co-authored medical research papers with him, and reviewed grants with him for the American Cancer Society. He is a gifted clinician and an accomplished researcher. He and his colleagues tell us that self-deception actually is a valuable personal coping tool—for a time—that allows us to "aspire to significance, strive for new knowledge, and yearn to make a lasting contribution to the world despite the certainty of our inevitable end." They remind us that we tend to overestimate benefits and underestimate costs when making our life plans, and we consequently make foolish decisions to embark on risky treatment pathways. This is referred to as the "planning fallacy."[10] The optimism that ensues helps us cope with the inevitability of death through denial. It follows that truthful conversations with doctors that acknowledge death can help patients understand their curability, are actually welcomed by patients, and do not squash hope or cause depression.

People have a bias toward optimism, but we must guard against optimism that is unrealistic.[11] The late Dr. Jane Weeks and her colleagues at the Dana Farber Cancer Institute at Harvard University asked nearly 1,200 patients with metastatic lung cancer or colorectal cancer whether they expected their treatment to cure them.[12] They found that the majority of patients with these conditions with a poor prognosis regardless of therapy felt that their treatment course was likely to "cure" them. Overall, more than two-thirds of patients with lung cancer and 81 percent of those with colorectal cancer did not report understanding that chemotherapy was not at all likely to cure their cancer. Somewhat surprisingly, educational level, functional status, and the patient's role in decision making were not associated with such inaccurate beliefs about chemotherapy.

The Harvard researchers concluded that many patients receiving chemotherapy for incurable cancers may not understand that chemotherapy is unlikely to be curative. This misunderstanding, in turn, could compromise their ability to make informed treatment decisions that are in agreement with their preferences. Physicians may be able to improve patients' understanding, but this may come at the cost of patients' satisfaction with them. The problem here may be the word *cure*.[10] To a patient with advanced disease, *cure* may mean something very different from eradication of all disease without return. To them, it may mean an end to pain or a hope for a better tomorrow with fewer incapacities. If patients actually have unrealistic expectations of a cure from a therapy that is administered with palliative intent, there is a serious problem of miscommunication by and with us physicians that we need to address.

Because we doctors are concerned about possible negative responses in our patients on hearing a poor prognosis, in many cases we do not tell patients who are dying that their disease is incurable. It is also possible that some physicians tell their patients about their poor prognoses, and the patients simply do not believe their doctors, or they do not understand. Observational studies have shown that two-thirds of doctors tell patients at the initial visit that they have an incurable disease, but only about a third actually state the prognosis—at any time.[13] It is not easy to tell patients that they are going to die, and most doctors choose not to do it. In fact, half of all patients with lung cancer have not heard any of their doctors use the word *hospice*.[14]

There are compelling data to recommend palliative care rather than treatment with curative intent in seriously ill patients. In a widely publicized study, researchers in multiple institutions randomly assigned patients with newly diagnosed metastatic and incurable lung cancer to receive either early palliative care with their standard oncologic care or standard oncologic care alone.[15] The researchers found that patients assigned to early palliative care had a better quality of life than did patients assigned to standard care. In addition, fewer patients in the palliative care group had depressive symptoms. Despite the fact that 20 percent fewer patients in the early palliative care group received aggressive end-of-life care, survival was nearly three months longer among patients receiving early palliative care alone. These data cast serious doubt on the value of aggressive treatment at the end of life for patients with incurable illness.

Patients may exhibit a number of responses upon receiving bad news.[16] These include sadness, anger, despair, gallows humor, and disbelief. If the treating physician doesn't address these responses properly, they can lead to anxiety, uncertainty, confusion, hopelessness, and a fear of losing control. Psychiatrists and clinical psychologists recommend that patients employ several strategies to deal with the distress they experience when receiving bad news. These include discussing the situation with a knowledgeable patient with the same situation, joining a support group, organizing and managing the parts of their lives that they can control, and making a clear treatment plan with their doctor.

Patients may also choose not to believe they are dying. When patients are given their actual prognosis, one-third or more will not admit that treatment will not cure them.[15] Patients with cancer have a very different perspective from those without such a diagnosis. In my experience it is possible to tell patients more effectively that they have a terminal illness through a sharing of information that enables them to plan better their remaining life. We oncologists can help patients understand by giving personalized facts. Nearly all patients want to know whether or not they can be cured, and the majority want to know their prognosis. Truthful conversations that acknowledge death help patients understand their curability, are welcomed by patients, and do not squash hope or cause depression.[10]

Divulging a Poor Prognosis

We doctors need help in breaking bad news. This is not one hard conversation for which we can muster our courage but rather a series of conversations that occur over time beginning with the recognition of the first existential threat to life. Experienced clinicians recommend stating the prognosis at the first visit, appointing someone in the office to ensure there is a discussion of advance directives, helping to schedule a hospice education appointment within the first three visits, and offering to discuss prognosis and coping ("What is important to you?") at each transition. This "best practices" model has allowed one large provider group to double patients' length of participation in hospice programs, maintain rates of survival, and decrease total costs.[17] Concurrent palliative care increases patients' knowledge of their prognosis, helps alleviate symptoms, reduces stress on caregivers, may improve survival, and lowers costs.[18]

These are not trivial issues. Chemotherapy near the end of life is still common, does not improve survival, and is one preventable reason why 25 percent of all Medicare funds are spent in the last year of life. Patients need truthful information in order to make good choices. If patients are offered truthful information—repeatedly—on what is going to happen to them, they can choose wisely. Most people want to live as long as they can, with a good quality of life, and then transition to a peaceful death outside the hospital. We have the tools to help patients make these difficult decisions. We just need both the courage and the incentives to use them.

Patients who died of hematologic malignancies (blood cancers) in one study used hospice about 25 percent of the time for a median of nine outpatient and six inpatient days.[19] This is better than the national rate of 2 percent for patients who died with hematologic malignancies, but it means that 75 percent of patients never experienced the benefits of hospice, including good symptom management, bereavement programs, less cost, and slightly lower mortality of the surviving spouse. Among cancer patients who were seriously ill enough to have been in the hospital during their last six months of life the average length of stay in hospice was just eight days among patients with an average age of seventy-eight years. Among these patients, 30 percent died in the hospital, 25 percent were in an intensive care unit in their last month of life, and only 54 percent ever used hospice. In addition to no referral, "late" referral to hospice means that patients may have less chance of having their end-of-life wishes known and honored, with more chance of dying with aggressive care or in the hospital rather than at home.

How Should We Then Die?
(with apologies to Francis A. Shaeffer[20])

Maintaining hope is an essential component of competent and compassionate oncology care,[21] yet hope has been criticized as having provided justification for paternalistic lies and half-truths to patients. British doctor Thomas Percival described physicians as ministers of hope and comfort to the sick. If the physician lies by withholding a truthful diagnosis or prognosis because she thinks the patient wants to be protected from the truth, she is being paternalistic. More than most other medical specialties, we oncologists understand the importance of hope. Our reluctance to disclose a grim prognosis may relate to our discomfort with putting odds on longevity, recurrence, and cure. We Americans value personhood, individual autonomy, and the power of thought to shape the course of our lives and the functioning of our bodies. Some of us oncologists say that controlling the facts we give to a patient is essential to maintaining or instilling an optimistic attitude. Although patients might find hope in the existence of God and eternal life, or in the accomplishment of some goal, this redirecting of hope away from therapies falsely believed to be curative is actually quite difficult to achieve. Our culture teaches us to believe in the possibility of miraculous cures, and the temptation to see hope in new therapies is great even when logic would dictate otherwise.

To achieve this redirection of hope, the psychological and spiritual resources of our patients and their families must be nurtured during a time when the patient is facing an illness that will end in death. Doctors using prognostic ambiguity or withholding information that is not specifically sought by a patient and her family may actually be employing an acceptable strategy for dealing with a dire prognosis. We physicians have a clear obligation to initiate discussions with our patients about their diagnoses, the specifics of treatment options and their side effects, and of their prognosis in general terms. We must also encourage patients and their family members to ask any question that is important for them and to provide multiple opportunities for such discussion. It is equally important that we physicians respect our patients' right to decline to receive additional details if they choose not to hear them.

When I administer chemotherapy to a patient with advanced cancer, the treatment carries with it the implication of hope. Because of the hope that accompanies any treatment, it is natural that it will foster optimism for many patients. We physicians who treat patients with life-threatening illness must go beyond simply responding to the patient's hope and become active participants in shaping more realistic expectations when disease progresses. Complete and total disclosure of all medical information may be the easiest course for most clinicians to follow, but we must be honest with our patients and use both common sense and human compassion. We have an obligation to promote hope in our patients, a central tenet and a guiding principle in medicine throughout the centuries. We can, nevertheless, disclose a grim prognosis with both compassion and sensitivity without being unnecessarily blunt.

Understanding Medical Futility to Control Costs

As we have seen, the costs of our care and the ways in which we die are not optimal in the United States today. What should we do about this? Can the challenging task of maintaining hope as we die be addressed, accompanied by hope of improving outcomes for patients who die? For the Christian physician, an affirmation of the promises of the gospel and the assurance of eternal life will engender hope in our patients.

Medical futility means that the proposed therapy should not be performed because available data show that it will not improve the patient's medical condition.[22] Futility "designates an effort to provide a benefit to a patient which reason and experience suggest is highly likely to fail and where rare exceptions cannot be systematically procured."[23] Futility can occur in several ways.[24] It can occur in process, in which a long and difficult course continues without any improvement. It can also occur in prognosis, when patients start treatment that has rarely or never proved useful in similar cases. And finally, it can occur in result, when treatment is technically successful but the resulting quality of life is undesirable.[25]

There is sometimes serious disagreement between physicians and families about the benefits to the patient of continued treatment when the patient or family believes that a treatment is effective but the treating doctor does not. Medical futility disputes are best avoided by strategies that optimize communication between physicians and their family members. Physicians must provide families with accurate, current, and frequent prognostic estimates. We must address the emotional needs of the family and try to understand the problem from the family's perspective.

We caregivers should advocate for and facilitate the provision of competent palliative care throughout the course of the illness. Physicians who care for the dying should support the drafting of laws that embrace futility considerations and should assist hospital boards and administrators in drafting hospital futility policies that both provide a fair process to settle disputes and embrace a defensible ethic of care.

Patients should share with their physicians what they know about their illness and discuss their expectations for the outcome of their treatment. They should also make a verbal contract with their physician about what they can accomplish together in their treatment. If doctors express a sense of futility about the disease and its outcome, the patient may feel helpless and become depressed. On the other hand, doctors who hide clinical realities from patients by using obscure medical terminology or by offering false hope in ineffective treatments or technology may allay a patient's anxiety for a time, but eventually the patient will feel that she has been deceived, leading to a lack of trust and a destruction of the therapeutic relationship.

As I have noted, when patients pursue medically futile treatments at the end of life, it is partly because of our poor communication with them. There are many studies that report how communication by physicians with patients can be improved.[26] We physicians must offer assistance to patients that guides them toward realistic expectations (e.g. "I will not have uncontrolled pain" or "I will be able to stay at home for as long as possible") and achievable goals such as participation in a clinical trial. Researchers note that it may be helpful to consider several points when determining if a treatment is medically futile.[27] These include asking, "What is the goal of the treatment in question?"

"What is the likelihood of achieving treatment goal(s)?" "What are the risks, costs, and benefits to the patient of pursuing the intervention, compared with alternatives?" "What are the individual needs of the patient?"

ASCO has issued a statement designed to help cancer patients and their doctors arrive at an agreed-upon plan of care that will achieve the patients' goals while avoiding futile and needlessly expensive care.[28] The components of this strategy include asking doctors to inform their patients about their prognosis and treatment options. Doctors should offer anticancer therapy when there is evidence to support its use in bringing about a meaningful clinical benefit. Interventions to improve the quality of a patient's life as well as its duration should be discussed throughout the course of the illness. Cancer doctors should discuss the likelihood and nature of the expected response, and the anticipated adverse effects and risks of any therapy. Direct costs in terms of time, toxicity, loss of alternatives, or possible financial effects should also be reviewed carefully. Finally, when cancer-specific treatment options are no longer available, doctors should encourage patients to transition to symptom-directed palliative care alone, where the goal is to minimize physical and emotional suffering and to ensure that patients with advanced cancer are given the opportunity to die with dignity and peace of mind.

AMA Seven Steps

The American Medical Association says seven steps should be included in a due process approach to declaring futility in specific cases.[29] These are listed in the endnotes to this chapter.[30]

Many states also have helpful web sites that can help patients and their families with issues at the end of life.[31] All clinicians who care for dying patients are to empower those patients to initiate realistic discussions of care options by providing more detailed information on prognosis, outcomes from standard interventions, and palliative care on clinic and patient-oriented web sites such as the National Cancer Institute's www.cancer.gov and ASCO's www.cancer.net.

What If It Were Your Mother?

After I describe a new treatment that I am recommending to a patient and her family I am meeting for the first time, I am often asked, "What would you do if this were your own mother?" The unstated implication is that I might recommend something different for her, as if I would reserve the best and most effective treatments only for a loved one of my own. Or that I might not choose to withdraw treatment from her in the face of medical futility.

We Christians who have illnesses that cannot be cured should resolve to die resolutely, with hope and dignity, knowing what comes after we die. We should die purposefully, but without enthusiasm (we need not want to die). We should die expectantly with assurance that God loves us, and we should die gracefully into his presence and into the whole company of angels. We should die unselfishly, able to answer the question about our own mothers with the conviction that we will not pursue the needless, the fruitless, or the futile treatment even for her. We should die mindful of the looming crisis of medical expenditures that are associated with no improvement in quality of life, and attentive to the real limitations of finite resources even in our very wealthy country.

Sally and I were dining at Jamie's 15 restaurant in London at the end of an eight-day theater and sightseeing trip in England with friends, parents, and alumni of Washington and Jefferson College, our son's alma mater. Throughout the week, we had gotten to know a dentist and his wife who is a breast cancer survivor. We had spoken several times during the week about the looming crisis in the American health care system. As we were discussing care for patients with incurable illness, Julie declared that there was a difference between what one can do and what one should do in circumstances of medical futility. Indeed there is, I agreed.

I had related to her the story of my mother's breast cancer and her resultant leukemia, and I explained that, rather than choosing to subject her to the demanding rigors of a second—almost certainly ineffective—induction therapy for her secondary leukemia, we elected, after much family discussion, to choose supportive care only and not to treat her leukemia again. Despite the protests of the Johns Hopkins oncologists caring for Mom, I made it very clear to my father and our family that survival would be extraordinary and unexpected in this situation of retreating a recurrent, chemotherapy-induced leukemia after failure of the initial induction regimen. The initial therapy had been exhausting and disorienting for Mother and resulted in a ten-week ordeal for her and my father. We were fearful that a second induction regimen would be even more taxing and dangerous for a sixty-three-year-old woman who, although medically well, was not physically fit and could die from treatment-related complications just as certainly as she was to die from the leukemia without chemotherapy. When we sent her home to her community hospital in Bethlehem, Pennsylvania, where she and her sisters had attended nursing school (and where my sister and I were born), she received the best supportive care possible. She died there very peacefully eleven days after she left Johns Hopkins. I would make the same decision today, years later, if I had to do it again. This is my answer to the often-asked question, "What would you do if it were your mother?" Futile care is not compassionate care, and we should neither recommend nor embrace it for our patients, cloaking it falsely as hope.

Recently, a patient of mine whom I had treated one year earlier for stage 2 breast cancer presented to me with a situation like the one we faced with my mother. She had a very aggressive monocytic leukemia with a very high leukemia blast cell count in her circulating blood. After referral to some of the senior hematologists in our practice, and after thoughtful discussion with her family, she decided not to receive treatment for her acute leukemia. She was sixty-eight years old, separated from her husband, but had a caring and engaged family who felt warmly toward her and loved her dearly. They all gathered in her room on the evening she was admitted to the hospital, and they were comfortable with her decision to receive only supportive care. She died quietly and peacefully without incident and with few symptoms within thirty-six hours of her presentation to me with her acute leukemia. I fully supported the decision she made with her family. Undeniably, the situation for her and for her family was tragic, and was as horrible as the situation I had found myself and my family in with my mother two decades earlier. No amount of love and concern for our families, however, can change the fact that our cherished family member is dying when no effective treatment exists anywhere in the world, and no treatment, no matter how sophisticated and no matter how famous the institution where it is delivered, can change the sad but undeniable reality that we are, at times, at the limits of our medical knowledge. No known treatment could save either my mother or my patient years later.

These are not situations in which to argue to do something, anything, to procure, by chance, some miraculous cure. Rather, I believe that if God wants to intervene miraculously in dire and desperate situations, he will do so without the aid of our medications. I am not advocating that we should tempt God, nor is this to say that we should abandon known remedies and rely on prayer or supplication alone in situations for which care is at hand. In my opinion, that would be both unethical and irresponsible. When we reach the limits of our knowledge, however, we should seek to provide solace and comfort at reasonable and conservative expense rather than to employ costly therapies known to be either ineffective or not proven to have any benefit in usual, similar, and representative clinical situations.

If the patient and her family insist on employing some sort of intervention in a clinical situation where successful treatment is unprecedented, a search for a clinical research trial, even with a Phase I drug that holds a very small chance of therapeutic success, should be undertaken. Families must recognize and acknowledge foremost in these situations that it is the patient who bears both the consequences and burdens of seeking treatment that is likely to be futile, and families should not insist on the patient's initiating and enduring such an ordeal if it will occur far from home in a location that makes it either inconvenient or impossible for the family to visit and regularly support the patient physically, spiritually, and emotionally. If the patient is not fully committed to the notion of therapy with curative intent, his wishes should be accepted and followed. In lieu of a clinical research trial, competent palliative and supportive care close to the patient's home is usually the most compassionate therapeutic plan. Families must recognize that treating their loved one in situations of medical futility does not connote or indicate greater care and concern for the patient. Such treatment is also no remedy for guilt held over long-standing and contentious family issues, nor will it serve to repair years of family strife and conflict. Futile therapy of the patient's life-threatening illness is not efficient or effective therapy of the family.

Futile therapy may also create an extremely difficult financial situation for the family after the patient's death. We expend far too large a portion of our health care dollars on treatments that are expensive, of minimal benefit—as measured by prolongation of life—and do not improve the quality of the lives of the patients we treat. As we noted earlier, there is a great deal of waste in US health care expenditures.[32] For example, we have new therapies for many illnesses in which the extension of overall survival with these treatments is often measured in days to weeks rather than months or years.[33] We need to ask ourselves whether giving such treatment is desirable given the minimal improvements in survival that we achieve. Increasingly in health care today, there are and will be trade-offs among an ever-expanding and ever more complex set of therapeutic options and alternatives. Not all of these treatments will be available to all patients in all clinical situations all of the time because of constraints of geography, travel expense, the medical condition of the patient, or the ability of the family to get the patient regularly and repeatedly to the sites where care is delivered.

Doctor, What if it Were Your Mother?

If we continue to expend finite resources on treatment for malignancies and other conditions for which we have poorly effective therapies and where we cannot demonstrate positive and beneficial outcomes, we will do so at the greater expense of not treating other individuals who have an excellent chance of survival given timely diagnosis and management of their illnesses. Money that might be spent on treatment of women with secondary acute leukemia that occurs as a result of their breast cancer treatment and for whom no curative therapy exists would be better spent on the rigorous and appropriate management of adult diabetes, for example, to avoid predictable complications such as cardiovascular disease, blindness, kidney failure, and limb amputations that occur with far greater frequency among patients with chronically inadequate control of their blood sugar levels.

As we baby boomers age, we and our children will need to become increasingly familiar with these choices and advocate regularly and more strongly for what we should do and not just for what we can do simply because we possess the technical competence to do so. Equally important, we must reach a social consensus that acknowledges there are things we should not do because the unrealized or unattainable benefits do not justify the costs that divert limited resources from more effective and efficient treatments that would be better employed for more common and curable diseases.

Most of us spend the majority of our adult lives denying the reality of our eventual deaths or denying the reality of the imminent death of an aging parent. This avoidance is, in my experience, the response to serious illness at the end of life by individuals who have never contemplated either seriously or thoughtfully their own mortality or that of the people they love. This avoidance results in what I shall call "substitutional intervention," i.e., treatments that, we hope, will further prolong and delay the inevitable death that occurs at the end of every life. This avoidance is a luxury we could never really afford and now certainly cannot indulge given the increasingly constrained economics of health care delivery. When we avoid contemplating our own mortality and the deaths of those we love because the thoughts are seemingly too painful, we simply create an existential dilemma from which we believe medicine can extricate us but that, in reality, it cannot. Medicine is a poor substitute for either theology or philosophy in wrestling with end-of-life issues, and futile treatment for incurable illnesses is a shabby surrogate for long, considered thought about therapeutic options and alternatives in medical situations where there is no hope of cure.

When Doctors are the Patients

It has been instructive for me to discuss these situations with my fellow oncologists who treat breast, lung, and colon cancers and hematologists who treat malignant lymphoma and leukemia. I have asked them what they would elect if *they* were the patient. Virtually uniformly they say they would not pursue aggressive therapy with curative intent for malignancies where survival is unprecedented (e.g., unresectable pancreas cancer or relapsed brain tumor). Rather, they profess that they would elect palliative options and hope to die peacefully without aggressive therapy. Admittedly, there may ultimately be neither atheists nor therapeutic nihilists in these speculative clinical foxholes, and it is possible that these physicians would pursue treatment in the same way that some of our patients and their families do when faced with these soul-wrenching situations, but I have observed them making such hard decisions for their own families and for themselves. They almost always elect the conservative option of less aggressive and more supportive approaches rather than rigorous treatments that have little or no objective data to support their use.

What I have also observed with some sadness and much surprise, however, is that some thoughtful and therapeutically conservative oncologists will often acquiesce to their patient's wishes and pursue therapies that they, themselves, would not elect. The cynic would argue that the motivation of these oncologists was greed, because those oncologists earn their incomes by administering therapy to their patients.[34] Greed may, in fact, motivate some oncologists, but I have rarely witnessed greed as the primary motivating factor in treatment recommendations. Far more often, in my experience, what we observe are the incessant demands and pleadings of patients and their families who simply cannot accept the notion that death is near, and they implore their physicians for one last fragment of hope. This is false hope, however, and, thankfully, some oncologists, neurologists, cardiologists, and internists have the necessary conversations that will avert needless and fruitless interventions.

We need to have more of these frank deliberations with our patients. It is not a sign of ignorance or failure if I tell my patient that cure is not possible when objectively it is not. I have had that conversation with countless patients with metastatic breast cancer during my career. I have simply said that theirs is a situation that can be controlled but not cured and that, eventually, they will die from their breast cancer. I have had that very painful conversation with a thirty-five-year-old mother of two children and many, many others. The reality is that after advanced breast cancer is treated with three or four chemotherapeutic regimens, the chance for further therapeutic benefit from additional treatment is very low, and palliative options should be sought. This recognition is neither cruel nor uncaring. Rather, I believe, the denial of palliative interventions is even crueler and more dishonest.

There are many reasons why a patient and her physician might continue treatment with curative intent beyond the point of clinical effectiveness. As we have noted, a patient may be uncomfortable with her own mortality and with the idea that sometimes doctors have limited ability to affect a cure because we have learned to believe that modern medicine can alleviate most ills. Second, the family may have unresolved issues of grief, obligation, or guilt that compel them to seek a cure where none exists. In addition, the doctor may be uncomfortable with the knowledge and the limits of medical science or may lack the social skills to navigate the treacherous environs of an excessively and unreasonably demanding family. In this age of super-specialization, the treating physician may regard the patient as a stranger and may feel uncomfortable with intimate discussions about imminent death. It is also likely, in many communities, that the resources and personnel to offer competent and compassionate palliative care do not exist, leaving both patient and family with only curative options for their care when, in reality, they desire something else, and they realize palliation would be appropriate were it available. A greater national focus on the universal provision of palliative and hospice care would remedy, in part, the therapeutic dilemma created for many patients and their families by our current health care system. Often, patients are unaware of all the options available to them, and better access to information would both facilitate decision making and promote more objective choices in the situations they confront at the end of life.

Strategies for People without Faith

What is the answer for the nonbeliever, the person whose worldview is not created by faith? We cannot allow selfishness or a lack of objectivity by the individual to bankrupt the rest of society. Futility and the use of ineffective, expensive treatment is not the antidote for a subjective negativism that sees palliation only in purchased "cures," especially when those marginal and imagined cures are both illusory and nonexistent. We must reject the idea that denying the use of futile treatment is equivalent to denying care. Make no mistake: care must always be provided with whatever means are available and as long as life prevails, but we must not confuse ineffective, yet technically competent, treatment with care and compassion. Again, it is not compassionate to do things known to be ineffective. Compassion equates to communicating honestly, relieving symptoms, maintaining hope (even if only in eternal life), and promising the provision of care until the last breath is drawn. We must surrender the notion that compassionate care can be purchased only at great price and that supportive care with relief of symptoms is somehow inferior to treatment with curative intent when you know that cure is not possible.

No patient has ever told me that they believed me to be incompetent or uncaring when I presented to them the notion that their cancer could be controlled but not cured. My patients simply want honesty and open engagement from me, and they reject fantasy notions about cures that do not exist. Patients will make informed and appropriate decisions if doctors present them with adequate and realistic information about their disease and its prognosis.

We Christians and all people of faith should be leaders in educating others in this process. We should look to the future, teaching the next generation by embracing palliative medicine and hospice care at the end of life. We should always approach our health care providers with questions about the quality of our care and about what technology and drug interventions can achieve and what they cannot. When the question is "Why should we die?" the answer at the end of useful interventions is "For this you were made..." May our dying be with the hope of ultimate comfort from the loving God who made us.

---

[1] Berwick, DM, Hackbarth AD. Eliminating waste in US health care. *JAMA* 2012;307:1513–1516.

[2] Stephen Brill reporting in *Time* magazine April 4, 2013.

[3] Smith TJ, Hillner BE. Bending the cost curve in cancer care. *N Engl J Med* 2011; 364:2060–2065.

[4] Mariotto AB, Yabroff KR, Shao Y, Feuer EJ, Brown ML. Projections of the cost of cancer care in the U.S.: 2010-2020. *J Natl Cancer Inst* 2011;103:117–128.

[5] Kelly RJ, Smith TJ. Delivering maximum clinical benefit at an affordable price: engaging stakeholders in cancer care. *Lancet Oncology* 2014;15:e112-118.

[6] Baselga J, Cortes J, Kim S-B, et al. Pertuzumab plus trastuzumab plus docetaxel for metastatic breast cancer. *N Engl J Med* 2012; 366:109–119.

[7] Cortes J, O'Shaughnessy J, Loesch D, et al. Eribulin monotherapy versus treatment of physician's choice in patients with metastatic breast cancer (EMBRACE): a phase 3 open-label randomised study. *The Lancet* 2011;377:914–923.

8. 1) Dow LA, Matsuyama RK, Ramakrishnan V, et al. Paradoxes in advance care planning: The complex relationship of oncology patients, their physicians, and advance medical directives. *J Clin Oncol* 2010;28:299–304; and 2) Von Roenn JH. Advance care planning: ensuring that the patient's voice is heard. *J Clin Oncol* 2013; 31:663–664.
9. Smith TJ, Longo TJ. Talking with patients about dying. *N Engl J Med* 2012;367:1651–1652.
10. Buehler, Roger; Griffin, Dale, & Ross, Michael (2002). "Inside the planning fallacy: The causes and consequences of optimistic time predictions." In Thomas Gilovich, Dale Griffin, & Daniel Kahneman (Eds.), *Heuristics and biases: The psychology of intuitive judgment*, pp. 250–270. Cambridge, UK: Cambridge University Press.
11. Crites J, Kodish E. Unrealistic optimism and the ethics of phase I research. *J Med Ethics* 2013;39:403–406.
12. Weeks JC, Catalano PJ, Cronin A, et al. Patients' expectations about effects of chemotherapy for advanced cancer. *N Engl J Med* 2012;367:1616–1625.
13. Kiely BE, Stockler MR, Tattersall MH. Thinking and talking about life expectancy in incurable cancer. *Semin Oncol* 2011;38:380–385.
14. Huskamp HA, Keating NL, Malin JL, et al. Discussions with physicians about hospice among patients with metastatic lung cancer. *Arch Intern Med* 2009;169:954–962.
15. Temel JS, Greer JA, Muzikansky A, et al. Early palliative care for patients with metastatic non–small-cell lung cancer. *N Engl J Med* 2010;363:733–742.
16. Baile WF, Beale EA. Giving bad news to cancer patients: matching process and content. *J Clin Oncol* 19;2001: 2575–2577.
17. Smith TJ, Temin S, Alesi ER, et al. American Society of Clinical Oncology provisional clinical opinion: the integration of palliative care into standard oncology care. *J Clin Oncol* 2012;30:880–887.
18. Hoverman JR, Cartwright TH, Patt DA, et al. Pathways, outcomes, and costs in colon cancer: retrospective evaluations in two distinct databases. *J Oncol Pract* 2011;7:Suppl:52s–59s.
19. Sexauer A, Cheng MJ, Knight L, et al. Patterns of hospice use in patients dying from hematologic malignancies. *J Pall Med* 2014, 17:195–199.
20. Shaeffer, Francis A. *How should we then live? The rise and decline of Western thought and culture*. Wheaton, IL: Crossway Books, 1976.
21. Kodish E, Post SG. Oncology and hope. *J Clin Oncol* 1995;13:1817–1822.

[22] Schneiderman LJ, Jecker NS, Jonsen AR. Medical futility: its meaning and ethical implications. *Ann Intern Med* 1990;112:949–954 Bernat JL. Medical futility: definition, determination, and disputes in critical care. *Neurocrit Care.* 2005;2:198-205.

[23] Jonsen AR, Siegler M, Winslade W. *Clinical Ethics: A Practical Approach to Ethical Decisions in Clinical Medicine.* New York: McGraw Hill, 2010.

[24] Jonsen AR. Futility (knowing when to stop): Intimations of futility. *Am J Med* 1994;96:107-109.

[25] Beauchamp TL, Childress JF. Conditions for overriding the prima facie obligation to treat. In Beauchamp TL, Childress JF, eds. *Principles of Biomedical Ethics.* 6th Edition. New York: Oxford University Press, 2009, 167-169 Lo B. Futile intervention. In Lo B, Ed. *Resolving ethical dilemmas. A Guide for Physicians.* 4th Ed. Philadelphia: Lippincott Williams & Wilkins, 2009, 61-66.

[26] DeLisser HM. How I conduct the family meeting to discuss the limitation of life-sustaining interventions: a recipe for success. *Blood* 2010;116;1648-1654; Barclay JS, et al. Communications strategies and cultural issues in the delivery of bad news. *J Palliat Med* 2007;10:958-977; Jacobsen J and Jackson VA. A communication approach for oncologists: understanding patient coping and communicating about bad news, palliative care, and hospice. *J Natl Compr Canc Net* 2009;7:475-480; Walling A, et al. Evidence-based recommendations for information and care planning in cancer care. *J Clin Oncol* 2008;26:3896-902.

[27] McCabe MS, Storm C. When doctors and patients disagree about medical futility. *J Oncol Pract* 2008;4:207–209.

[28] Peppercorn JM, Smith TJ, Helft PR, et al. American Society of Clinical Oncology Statement: Toward individualized care for patients with advanced cancer. *J Clin Oncol* 2011;29:755-760.

[29] www.ama-assn.org//ama/pub/physician-resources/medical-ethics/code-medical-ethics/opinion2037.page

[30] American Medical Association Seven Steps to a due process approach to declaring medical futility in the face of disagreement between physician and patient

1. Earnest attempts should be made in advance to deliberate over and negotiate prior understandings between patient, proxy, and physician on what constitutes futile care for the patient, and what falls within acceptable limits for the physician, family, and possibly also the institution.

2. Joint decision-making should occur between patient or proxy and physician to the maximum extent possible.
3. Attempts should be made to negotiate disagreements if they arise, and to reach resolution within all parties' acceptable limits, with the assistance of consultants as appropriate.
4. Involvement of an institutional committee such as the ethics committee should be requested if disagreements are irresolvable.
5. If the institutional review supports the patient's position and the physician remains unpersuaded, transfer of care to another physician within the institution may be arranged.
6. If the process supports the physician's position and the patient/proxy remains unpersuaded, transfer to another institution may be sought and, if done, should be supported by the transferring and receiving institution.
7. If transfer is not possible, the intervention need not be offered.

© American Medical Association 1995-2014. All rights reserved.

[31] www.portal.state.pa.us/portal/server.pt/community/directory_of_services/4984/advance_directives_for_health_care?qid=39798655&rank=8

[32] Berwick DM, Hackbarth AD. Eliminating waste in US health care. JAMA 2012;307:1513-1516.

[33] Consider, for example, Smith TJ, Longo DL. Talking with patients about dying. *N Engl J Med* 2012; 367:1651-1652 Weeks JC, Catalano PJ, Cronin A, et al. Patients' expectations about effects of chemotherapy for advanced cancer. *N Engl J Med* 2012;367:1616-1625

[34] Brawley, Otis W with Goldberg, Paul. *How we do harm.* New York: St. Martin's Press, 2011

19

Some Final Thoughts on Communicating Hope

> Love does not delight in evil but rejoices with the truth. It always protects, always trusts, always hopes, always perseveres. Love never fails.
> —1 Corinthians 13:6–8

The medical literature demonstrates a positive association between the depth of religious belief or practices and mental or physical health outcomes. Hundreds of research studies and dozens of review articles reflect positively on the association between spirituality and physical and mental health outcomes from disease.[1] Research demonstrates that more than three-fourths of patients believe their physicians should address spiritual issues as part of their medical care. Patients can and should expect their physicians to respect their beliefs and to talk about spiritual concerns in a respectful and caring manner. Although nearly 80 percent of Americans believe in the power of God or prayer to improve the course of illness, and nearly two-thirds want their physicians to address spiritual issues, fewer than 10 percent of the physicians actually do so. Nearly half of inpatients want their physicians to pray with them, yet these patients report that their physicians rarely discussed spiritual matters. In the past, only 5 percent of physicians reported that religious and spiritual issues were addressed in their training.[2] Now, most medical schools provide training in addressing faith and spiritual issues with patients.

Physicians need to learn to take a spiritual history that identifies religious or spiritual needs in their patients and then coordinates the resources required to meet those needs. Many physicians feel uncomfortable addressing the topic of religion, and many patients may not expect a physician to ask even though such questions might be welcomed. Simply taking a spiritual history is often an intervention nevertheless.[3] Frequently, all that is necessary is to listen to the patient's responses, providing presence and support rather than demonstrating expertise in religious matters. Although providing spiritual advice or direction is probably best left to a chaplain or to the patient's clergy, the spiritual history should not necessarily be deferred to others. When the physician asks these questions, it signals to the patient that the physician cares about the patient's sources of hope and meaning during illness. When religion is what gives meaning, purpose, and hope, patients are often comforted by sharing their beliefs with their physicians. Spiritual counselors tell us that when there are religious doubts or anxieties present, sharing these feelings with a caring, accepting physician may help a patient with resolution.

We are cautioned that care must be taken that the nonreligious physician does not underestimate the importance of the patient's belief system. We "religious physicians" who believe differently from our patient must not impose our beliefs onto the patient at this time of special vulnerability. In both cases, the principle of respect for the patient should transcend the ideology of the physician.[4] I have always taken this approach.

Published guidelines can assist physicians in the consideration of religious issues.[5] Physicians are told that we may enter such a dialogue, but we are not obligated to do so. Our dialogues must be at the invitation of the patient, not imposed by us, and we must be open and nonjudgmental in claiming that our beliefs are personally helpful. We cannot, of course, claim that we have the "ultimate truth," and the guiding principle should be that we follow the foundational Hippocratic principle to "do no harm." In all cases, the purpose of our dialogues should be burden-lifting and not burden-producing.

Tools are available to help cancer doctors provide better data about the risks and benefits of treatment by sharing anticipated response rates, chances of cure (always near zero for patients with metastatic solid tumors), and side effects; discussing transitional care to hospice; and allowing patients and families to make informed decisions and to maintain hope.[6] Such tools help reset expectations and help patients, families, and providers accept the transition to non-chemotherapy palliative care. Sadly, however, many oncologists do not have these skills.[7] This is something we need to change in American health care. Changing it will require more education of physicians who care for patients at the end of their lives. It will also require changes in our health care system so that monetary incentives are provided to physicians to avoid using care that is either futile or unnecessary. These payments could be made from the millions of dollars that we can save by avoiding care that improves neither the quality nor the duration of the life of a patient who is dying.

Handouts are also available from the American Academy of Family Physicians and other organizations that explain to patients in lay language what spirituality is and how it can be related to health. They also provide suggestions to improve spiritual health and inform patients what their doctors need to know about their spiritual beliefs.[8]

Truthful conversations that acknowledge the reality of death help patients understand their curability, are welcomed by patients, and do not squash hope or cause depression as is widely believed.[9] When doctors are giving bad news to patients, they should (1) state the prognosis at the first visit, (2) appoint someone in the office to ensure there is a discussion of advance directives, (3) help patients schedule a meeting about hospice visit within the first three visits, and (4) offer to discuss prognosis and coping. This approach has doubled patients' length of participation in hospice programs, maintained rates of survival, and decreased total costs.[10] Concurrent palliative care increases knowledge of prognosis, helps alleviate symptoms, reduces stress on caregivers, may improve survival, and has been shown to lower costs. As we have noted, these are not trivial issues. Unfortunately, chemotherapy near the end of life is still common, does not improve survival, and is one preventable reason why 25 percent of all Medicare funds are spent in the last year of life.

Communication skills are critical to a successful and competent medical oncologist, but, as I have noted, few of us have been trained in these skills. Fortunately, programs are being developed to impart these abilities to cancer specialists in training.[11] My former colleague Dr. Robert Arnold at the University of Pittsburgh and others studied both oncologists and their patients with advanced cancer to learn about their communication with each other.[12] I was pleased to be included as one of the physicians in their research. They concluded that both oncologists and patients need to work to create an alliance that allows patients to express their emotions. They determined that this happens, in part, when oncologists respond empathically when patients express negative emotions. We oncologists, despite our confidence in addressing emotions, probably need more training to recognize feelings in our patients and to learn how to respond to patients' concerns. Patients too, they decided, may need to learn how to express their emotions more directly so that we oncologists are given the opportunity to respond appropriately. This requires that we spend more time listening and talking and, perhaps, less time diagnosing and treating medically our patients with advanced illness.

When doctors give bad news, it is stressful both for them and their patients. Physicians may distance themselves from difficult clinical situations and avoid discussing life-threatening aspects of the patient's disease. This distancing will often lead to distrust of the physician by the patient and her family. To protect themselves emotionally and psychologically, patients may engage in wishful thinking about their illnesses and may harbor unrealistic expectations about the outcome of their disease. It is also not uncommon for patients to hide fearful and pessimistic thoughts from their doctors.[13]

Medical ethicists describe four models that define the care we clinicians provide for types and stages of illnesses that carry different expectations for both their duration and the outcomes affected by treatment.[14] When a patient has a serious but acute condition, a cure is not only possible but also expected, and the model for serious illness applies. When the illness is chronic, on the other hand, and we expect inexorable deterioration in the patient's quality of life and progression of disease, our treatment provides alleviation of symptoms without the expectation of cure. In these conditions, treatment may be delivered over a very long period of time, and a model for chronic conditions is then most appropriate. In a similar way, conditions that require ongoing palliative care for patients who are not hospitalized employ a model of continual treatment and active involvement of both the patient and the health care provider. A final model applies when there is a low probability of cure such as when we treat metastatic cancer.[15]

My Goals as an Oncologist When Providing Care at the End of Life

As I have emphasized repeatedly in this book, my goal and overriding principle when caring for patients with cancer is to provide as much information as the patient and her family desire. I attempt to keep both the patient and her caregivers involved in the process of treatment and the decision making that occurs throughout our time together. I always strive to present the facts using nontechnical and layman's language. I also endeavor to avoid what I call *"Onco-hubris,"* a behavioral tendency of oncologists that holds that we are the keepers of special knowledge and that our opinions should be both respected and unquestioned. This lofty and egotistical view is a certain recipe for clinical disaster and does not respect the autonomy of our patients. It can be avoided by speaking plainly, by not condescending, and by respecting the ability of all patients and their families, no matter how limited their education or experience, to make rational and informed decisions when provided with clear and objective data. These principles are listed below.

Guidelines for Interactions with the Sick and Dying

- Promise to be with the patient until the end.
- Deliver a prognosis that illness will end in death by explaining that we do not have a lot of time left together.
- Define realistic expectations for the remaining days.
- Spend time listening to the dying and the suffering and elicit their expectations.
- Allow the dying to grieve for the losses they are experiencing: loss of self; loss of vocation and a sense of self-value; loss of family, friends, and relationships; and, finally, loss of future. Encourage mourning for the loss of what will never be.
- Engage the dying in making plans for their death and allow them to direct as many decisions as possible.
- Endeavor to remain honest in the information delivered, and strive to keep clinical expectations reasonable.

As described above, we must know when to change our mode of care from one with curative intent to one of dealing with chronic symptoms and maintaining good performance status. We must also be fully aware of when to transition finally to a palliative-care mode where our goal is to control symptoms for as long as possible.

As I explained earlier, it is both necessary and our obligation to explore spiritual concerns whenever they arise, and to make timely and appropriate referrals to clergy and spiritual advisers who are trained and competent in the provision of these services.

We must also pursue with greater diligence the completion of advance directives by our patients who are facing and suffering through life-threatening illness. The completion of these documents provides clarity for them and their families, removes ambiguity and uncertainty for family members and loved ones, and provides a clear path during the patient's final days when they may be unable to communicate their wishes.

POLST (Physician Orders for Life Sustaining Therapies) is an intervention that requires a clinician to discuss and document a patient's advance care wishes.[16] It is a physician's order that contains a patient's choices about the nature and extent of life-sustaining procedures that they may wish to have done or omitted. It is signed not only by the doctor but also by the patient or her surrogate. Currently, not all states recognize POLST orders as binding. It is, however, a durable document that, when used, has been shown to make treatment consistent with patients' wishes 90 percent of the time.

In my clinical encounters with the dying, I respond to suffering by making the promise that I will be with the patient until the end. I deliver a prognosis that illness will end in death by explaining that we do not have a lot of time left together, and that we must define realistic expectations for the remaining days. Those of us who care for the dying and the suffering must spend a great deal of time listening to them, and we must allow them to grieve for the losses they are experiencing: their loss of self, loss of vocation and a sense of self-value; loss of family, friends, and relationships; and, finally their loss of the future, what for them will never be. We must be patient and take time to hear what our patients are saying to us. I once had a patient with advanced breast cancer say that I was always in a hurry, and that she wanted another oncologist to provide her care. I made a conscious effort to slow down and listen to her, and we restored our therapeutic relationship. We need to engage the dying in making plans for their death and allow them to direct as many decisions as are possible. In all my discussions with the dying, I attempt to remain honest in the information that I deliver and strive to keep clinical expectations realistic.

The Physician at the Memorial Service

I have made it a habit over my professional career to attend the memorial services of the patients with whom I have grown close during their illnesses. Rare physicians have advocated over the years that it is valuable for physicians to attend the funerals of their patients. Some doctors have explained that it gives families an opportunity to talk about their experiences surrounding the death of their loved one. In addition, the presence of the physician who cared for the patient adds credibility to the sense of worth that family members gather about the deceased. Perhaps most important, family members regard the physician's attendance as a demonstration of caring for the person who died. The presence of the doctor signals that he views his patient as more than a business client, consumer, or scientific curiosity with an unusual disease. My presence says that the patient had value to me as a human being.[17] My attendance also says to the community that the lives of my patients are important to me, even in death. Their families are also important to me. I value and respect their losses in the passing of the one they entrusted to my care.

Looking Toward the Future

If we do not make the required changes in our health care system within the next decade, we will bankrupt the entire system as we 70 million baby boomers age and needlessly consume resources without improving our lives as we die. This will ultimately worsen the quality of the lives of our children and grandchildren and incur debts for them for many, many years to come. Our hope lies in our ability to make thoughtful and rational decisions for ourselves so that we do not needlessly burden our heirs with a legacy derived from our hopelessness. We need not be so cynical. We merely need, rather, to embrace our finitude and make informed choices so that we may die with hope for future generations who will inherit the consequences of our choices. Let us make those choices out of hope and not out of fear, out of thoughtfulness and clear thinking rather than out of dread and compulsive over-consumption of finite and precious health care resources.

Doctors and patients need to work collectively to develop a plan for hope in reforming our health care system. We need to work on returning to patient-centered care that focuses on what patients need rather than on what their doctors and their families may want. We need to focus on the difference between knowledge and hope and learn how knowledge of what is futile can actually engender hope. We all need to embrace the reality of the end of life: that it is inevitable and that it will come for all of us. For all of us there will come a time when medicine can no longer provide a solution to our suffering. We need to work fervently to avoid false hope, but at the same time to sustain hope even when survival is unprecedented—not hope for cure or miraculous recovery but hope for a peaceful death.

There is a role for anger and the will to fight because life is precious, and we must love it. But there is also a time for surrendering without giving up, for clarifying goals and finding peace. We need to learn how to review the life milestones and commitments of the dying, and we need to learn better to say goodbye without avoiding those emotionally demanding yet rewarding conversations. When the time comes, we must acknowledge that the end is at hand, that life has many disappointments along with its many joys, and that dying honorably and thoughtfully is what we all must aspire to do. Death will come violently and needlessly for some, far before the desires of a full life are realized. I am painfully aware of that harsh reality. But when the end comes and no more can be done by medicine and human intervention, let us go quietly and in peace. Although we may rage against the dying of the light, we must go gentle into that good night.

---

[1] Larimore WL. Providing basic spiritual care for patients: should it be the exclusive domain of pastoral professionals? *Am Fam Phys* 2001;63:36-41.

[2] Shafranske EP, Malony HN. Clinical psychologists' religious and spiritual orientations and their practice of psychotherapy. *Psychotherapy* 1990;27:72-78.

[3] Koenig HG. Spiritual assessment in medical practice. *Am Fam Phys* 2001;63:30-33.

[4] McCormick TR. "Spirituality and medicine." University of Washington School of Medicine. *http://depts.washington.edu/bioethx/topics/spirit.html* (Accessed September 13, 2014)

5. Foster DW. Religion and Medicine: The Physician's Perspective. In Marty ME, Vaux KL, eds. *Health/Medicine and the Faith Traditions.* Philadelphia: Fortress Press, 1982, 245-270.
6. Smith TJ, Dow LA, Virago E, Khatcheressian J, Lyckholm LJ, Matsuyama R. Giving honest information to patients with advanced cancer maintains hope. *Oncology* 2010;24:521-525.
7. Jackson VA, Mack J, Matsuyama R, et al. A qualitative study of oncologists' approaches to end-of-life care. *J Palliat Med* 2008;11:893-906.
8. American Academy of Family Physicians. Spirituality and health. *Am Fam Physician* 2001;63:89.
9. Mack JW, Smith TJ. Reasons why physicians do not have discussions about poor prognosis, why it matters, and what can be improved. *J Clin Oncol* 2012;30:2715-2717.
10. Smith TJ et al. Ibid.
11. Back AL, Arnold RM, Baile WF, et al. Faculty development to change the paradigm of communication skills teaching in oncology. *J Clin Oncol* 2009;27:1137-1141.
12. Pollak KJ, Arnold RM, Jeffreys AS, et al. Oncologist communication about emotion during visits with patients with advanced cancer. *J Clin Oncol* 2007;25:5748-5752.
13. Baile WF, Beale EA. Giving bad news to cancer patients: matching process and content. *J Clin Oncol* 19;2001: 2575-2577.
14. Jonsen AR, Siegler M, Winslade WJ. *Clinical Ethics.* New York: Macmillan, 1982. Jonsen AR, Siegler M, Winslade W. *Clinical Ethics: A Practical Approach to Ethical Decisions in Clinical Medicine.* New York: McGraw Hill, 2010.
15. Jonsen AR, Siegler M, Winslade WJ. Ibid, 1982.
16. Bomba PA, Vermilyea D. Integrating POLST into palliative care guidelines: a paradigm shift in advance care planning in oncology. *J Natl Compr Canc Net* 2006;4:819-829 www.polst.org (Accessed September 13, 2014)
17. Irvine, P. The attending at the funeral. *N Engl J Med* 1985;312:1704-1705.

Acknowledgments

No book would be possible without the help and generous support of a number of individuals.

I would like to thank my late father, the Reverend Victor G. Vogel Jr., for the thoughtful and insightful guidance and counsel he gave to me throughout my entire life. His direction was central to my early spiritual developmental. He introduced me to the richness and depth of Holy Scripture and armed me for the long and, at times, arduous journey that has been my career. I thank him, too, for our many discussions throughout my life related to the topics reviewed and discussed in this book. He espoused and lived his "resurrection theology" and offered it as sustenance to the many sick and dying individuals whom he visited and cared for during his more than forty years in the parish ministry. His was the beacon that always brought me back to my spiritual center.

I thank my wife, Sally, for her constant presence and support for more than forty years of our lives together and for her tolerance of my many absences during my academic career. They were both frequent and protracted, and she willingly shared me with that selfish mistress, medicine, through our training and our years of clinical practice. As a pediatrician, she was an ever-present sounding board for the many challenges and vexations of my early clinical career. She was an ideal mother for our two children, whose growth, development, and vocational success would not have been possible without her loving and attentive care. She permitted me to pursue the dark and lonely experience that is writing, and I am forever grateful for her loving gifts.

Our children, Heather and Christiaan, were exceptionally accepting of my frequent absences during their developmental years, and by God's grace, they seem no worse for wear. They were a delight for Sally and me as they grew up in our home, and they are the true jewels in my crown of life. I cannot adequately express my pride in them or my love for them. They have challenged and questioned me in ways that, I hope, have made my ideas more complete and comprehensible to others. They have both inspired me more than they can know.

I have had a number of pastors who have guided and shepherded me over many decades. I owe thanks to all of them, including H. Daehler Hayes; Lyle Harper and his wife, Dotti; Jerry Wicklein and his wife, Pam; Russ Ward and his wife, Lilly Wray; Thomas Hill and his wife, Janet; Douglas Meyer; Scott Endress; Keefe Cropper; Robert Heppenstall; Chris Taylor; George Wirth; and William S. Henderson. I also owe special thanks to Anglican priest Owen Vigeon and to pastor William Petry, who were kind enough to read the manuscript and to offer very helpful criticism and corrections. The Reverend Keith Brown was a colleague of my father and a mentor and resource to me in a time of crisis in our local church congregation in Pittsburgh. He taught me patience, forgiveness, and forbearance along with a large dose of humility when I needed it most. For his many gifts, I am very thankful. His lessons were life changing for me.

Special thanks to Judy and Ted Sentz in Summersville, West Virginia, who warmly received Sally and me as two very young and green physicians straight out of our residency training into their community, their home, and their church. They made us feel welcome, and celebrated with us the joyous event of the birth of our daughter, Heather. We will always hold a special place in our hearts for the many kindnesses they showed to us during our brief but happy years in their town. A similar warm thanks goes to Tim and Peggy Hugus, who have been dear friends to us for more than thirty years and have supported us through many of our life transitions. Their faith and friendship have endeared them to Sally and me and have been a joy and comfort to us, both in challenging times and in times of celebration.

I would also like to thank Dr. William J. Carl, president of the Pittsburgh Theological Seminary, and Dr. Ron Cole-Turner, H. Parker Sharp Professor of Theology and Ethics at the school, for their advice and friendship. I also thank Rebecca Cole-Turner for her spiritual light, her thoughtful discussions, and her uplifting correspondence over the years.

I extend warm thanks to both Kathi Pater and Adrienne Weiss, who provided expert administrative assistance to me during my many years at the University of Pittsburgh Cancer Institute and the Magee-Womens Hospital. They helped me juggle multiple demands on my time that were both academic and clinical, and I am forever grateful for their assistance with schedules, travel arrangements, meeting agendas and coordination, and much correspondence. I also thank them for their listening ears and gentle encouragement during the process of writing this book.

I am very grateful for many willing patients who thought with me, discussed the concepts for this book, and shared their hopes and concerns: Sister Paula Beiter; Julie Benner; Margaret Dewald; Julia Huntington; Karen Storm; Brenda Eck and her husband, Steve; and Paula Keller and her husband, Chris. Their honesty and encouragement about my ideas for this book were invaluable. I extend very special thanks to Patty Easton for her superb critique of the manuscript and to and her husband, Richard, for his friendship and encouragement.

I also owe special thanks to Dr. Otis Brawley, chief medical officer of the American Cancer Society, who gave me the opportunity to act briefly as the national vice president for research for the ACS. In that role, I was afforded time to learn and think about cancer as a public health problem and to consider it outside the confines of the examination room and the hospital bed. It was there that I thought seriously for the first time about palliative approaches to end-of-life care. I had the opportunity to hear perspectives from clinicians and cancer survivors across the country and to think about approaches that might bring improvement to our care for cancer patients in their final months of life. Dr. Jerome Yates, my predecessor at the ACS, was instrumental in bringing me into the organization, and his insight and unique perspectives have been invaluable to me over the years. I would also like to thank Dr. J. Leonard Lichtenfeld, deputy chief medical officer at the ACS, whom I have known for forty years, for his special insights into cancer as a social problem and for his special appreciation of cancer as an often daunting clinical challenge. His advice and friendship have been extremely useful to me for many years.

Brad Richards, JD, partner at Hayes and Boone, LLP in Houston, Texas, and his wife, Amy, shared in discussions with me about the ideas in the book, and I am grateful for their time and insight.

Several nurses have assisted me greatly by providing expert oncologic care to my patients, and have been listening ears and faithful partners with me in ushering many women through the final days. Susan Wood, Elizabeth Mcdermott, and Lori Sabotchick will always have my deepest respect for their professionalism, their caring, and their friendship toward both me and our patients. I have learned a great deal from each of them, and it has been an honor to work so closely with them. I would not have been able to solve many of the clinical problems we confronted without their caring and compassion for our patients. They helped me guide many patients through the process of dying with both faith and objectivity. For that I am forever in their debt, and our patients and their families will be forever grateful.

I have also learned a great deal from John Gerdis, PhD, and Charlotte Collins, PhD, who have been reliable and resourceful colleagues in the psychological care of many women who were challenged emotionally and spiritually in dealing with their cancers. Their gentle expertise has eased the suffering for scores of my patients, and we are in their debt.

Bill and Linda Petry have been special friends in a time of transition, and Sally and I both thank them for showing us true Christian hospitality.

My family, including my sister and brother, Louise (a.k.a. "Louie") and Tim, and many others have sustained me through a sometimes tortuous and burdensome journey with patience and sustenance that have ushered me through trying and difficult times. I have seldom acknowledged how dear they have been to me and how impossible my career would have been without their patient and abiding love and care.

For the countless patients and their families who have permitted me to share with them their joys and sorrows, their celebrations and their grief, their hopes and their faith, I am forever grateful. You were a blessing to me in more ways than you can ever know.

Biography

Dr. Victor Vogel is a medical oncologist who has been taking care of women with breast cancer and doing clinical research in breast oncology for 30 years. He is currently Director of Breast Medical Oncology/Research at the Geisinger Health System in central Pennsylvania. He is a graduate of the Temple University School of Medicine and the Johns Hopkins Bloomberg School of Public Health. He was the Deputy Director of the Community Clinical Oncology Program research base at the University of Texas M. D. Anderson Cancer Center in the mid-1980s and 1990s. He was a member of the Steering Committee for the National Surgical Adjuvant Breast and Bowel Program (NSABP) Breast Cancer Prevention Trial and was protocol chairman for the NSABP STAR trial that enrolled more than 19,000 women in the US and Canada. He also served on the NSABP Board of Directors for 10 years. For 10 years he was also a member of the Data and Safety Monitoring Committee of the Women's Health Initiative of the National Institutes of Health, appointed by Health and Human Services Secretary Bernadine Healy. He was a member of the Central Institutional Review Board (IRB) of the National Cancer Institute (NCI) and served a mini-sabbatical in the Division of Cancer Prevention on an Interagency Personnel Agreement in 2003-2004. He was a member of the Grants Council at the American Cancer Society

(ACS), served on grant review study sections at both ACS and NCI, and was National Vice President for Research at the ACS from 2009-2010.

At the University of Pittsburgh Medical School he was chairman of the oncology Institutional Review Board and a member of the university's IRB Executive Committee. He has served as principal investigator on a number of investigator-initiated and cooperative group protocols at all of the institutions where he has held appointments during the three decades of his clinical and academic career. He is currently the Director of Breast Medical Oncology/Research for the Geisinger Health System in central Pennsylvania, one of the country's largest integrated health systems.

Dr. Vogel has personally sustained life-threatening and disabling injuries and illnesses. He endured the death of his mother when he was a young oncologist and wrestled with the limits of medical care. A lifelong Christian, he has struggled with the challenges of answering questions about suffering and death for his patients, his family, and his friends. He is an ordained Presbyterian elder and a member of the Board of Directors of the Pittsburgh Theological Seminary. He has edited two medical textbooks, is the author of hundreds of professional articles and editorials, was a medical school professor for 22 years, and has traveled and lectured on four continents. He has appeared on national news broadcasts and has been quoted in the New York Times. He has been married for 37 years to a pediatrician, is the father of two children, and has two grandchildren.